FAT

BOOKS BY KIT REED

Novels
TIGER RAG
CRY OF THE DAUGHTER
ARMED CAMPS
THE BETTER PART
AT WAR AS CHILDREN
MOTHER ISN'T DEAD SHE'S ONLY SLEEPING

Short Stories
MR. DA V AND OTHER STORIES

Juvenile
WHEN WE DREAM

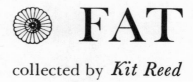

FAT

collected by *Kit Reed*

THE BOBBS-MERRILL COMPANY, INC.
Indianapolis • New York

ISBN 0-672-51979-8
Library of Congress catalog card number 73-22670
Designed by Jacques Chazaud
Manufactured in the United States of America

First printing

This book is for all thin fat people, but especially for a cousin of mine who once lost 115 pounds

ACKNOWLEDGEMENTS

"The Three Fat Women of Antibes," copyright © 1933 by W. Somerset Maugham, from *The Complete Short Stories of W. Somerset Maugham.* Reprinted by permission of Doubleday Company, Inc. and the Literary Executor of W. Somerset Maugham and William Heinemann Ltd.

"Fat Man," by George Garrett, from *Abraham's Knife and Other Poems*, copyright © 1959, 1961 by George Garrett.

"The Ordeal of Fats Goldberg," by Calvin Trillin. Reprinted by permission; © 1971 Calvin Trillin. Originally in *The New Yorker.*

"Starting on Monday," by Judith Viorst, copyright © 1971 by Judith Viorst. From *People and Other Aggravations.* With permission of the author and Thomas Y. Crowell Co., Inc.

"The Echo and the Nemesis," by Jean Stafford, reprinted with the permission of Farrar, Straus & Giroux, Inc. from *The Collected Stories of Jean Stafford*, copyright © 1950, 1969 by Jean Stafford. Note copyright © 1974 by Jean Stafford.

"The Food Farm," by Kit Reed, copyright © 1974 by Kit Reed.

"Fat City," by Burr Snider. Reprinted by permission of International Famous Agency and Burr Snider. Copyright © 1973 by Esquire Inc. First appeared in *Esquire* magazine.

From *The Life and Times of William Howard Taft* by Henry F. Pringle, copyright © 1939 by Henry F. Pringle. Reprinted by permission of Holt, Rinehart and Winston, Inc.

"Boule de Suif," by Guy de Maupassant, translated by Carl A. Viggiani, translation copyright © 1974 by Carl A. Viggiani.

"Fat Girl," by Brendan Gill, reprinted by permission: © 1970 *The New Yorker Magazine, Inc.*

"Obesity and Eating," by Stanley Schachter, copyright © 1968 by the American Association for the Advancement of Science. Reprinted from *Science Magazine* vol. 161, pp. 751-756 (23 Aug. 1968), with permission of the author.

"Thin Fat People," by Hilde Bruch. Chapter 11 of *Eating Disorders*, by Hilde Bruch, copyright © 1973 by Basic Books, Inc., Publishers, New York.

EDITOR'S NOTE

As all good eaters know, fat collects. When I began work on this book some four years ago, I had a nucleus of four or five pieces. As soon as I announced I was in the FAT business, everybody I knew began coming up with suggestions, and because of their interest, the collection grew rapidly.

In addition to the people represented in the table of contents, I'd like to thank Richard Wilbur, Richard Slotkin, F. D. Reeve, Sam Pottle, Judith Merril, A. S. Wensinger, John Crigler, Richard Wood, Adrian Mitchell, Phyllis Rose, Clem Vose, Nancy Campbell and all the people who began bubbling with ideas when they heard about FAT. I'd also like to thank Joan Roseman of Brandt and Brandt, Don Erickson of *Esquire*, Jane Ogle of *Harper's Bazaar*, Joan Jurale and other staff members at the Olin Library at Wesleyan University; Robert G. Campbell, M.D.; William G. Shipman, Ph.D.; Dr. William Asher and Dominic Crolla of the American Society of Bariatric Physicians, and especially Carl Brandt, for his continuing enthusiasm for the project, and Betty Kelly of Bobbs-Merrill Inc., who has helped me bring the book to publication.

I'd like to give special thanks to my husband the artist, Joseph Reed, and to Ellen Gates D'Oench, for her matchless research and patient persistence in the matter of obtaining reprint rights. With added thanks to John Reed, my proofreader.

TABLE OF CONTENTS

FAT

INTRODUCTION

I have at least two friends who claim to have said it first: "Inside every thin person, there's a fat one screaming. . ."

I know it is true of me.

In the grammar school I went to, there were several dread days which are still seared on my memory. One was the day in the fourth grade when the teacher took us into the cloak room, one by one, and riffled our hair with the tip of her ruler; somebody, who remained nameless, had turned up at school with lice; maybe the contagion had spread; for the time being, we were all suspect. As we waited our turns outside the cloak room, we nine-year-olds exchanged looks of suspicion and mutual guilt.

Listen, it isn't me.

Then, with eyes narrowed:

I bet it's you.

We never heard any more about it so I guess it wasn't any of us, but we understood each other from that moment: when in doubt, cast the first stone.

Which laid the groundwork for all the dread days to follow: the discovery of the first bosom (never mind whose), the first moustache; Oral English days, and the most terrible day of all: the day in the seventh grade when they decided to move the scales into the classroom and weigh everybody. The nurse did the weighing and called out the figures to the teacher, who wrote them down. Which is how I ended up being the fattest kid in the class.

I must have seen it coming; I remember pointing to a pudgy red-headed kid and whispering, a diversionary tactic; Betty Jean Hoffman and I exchanged giggles: hee hee

hee. I already knew it wasn't going to work. First we had to line up alphabetically and then, right out there in front of everybody, we had to step on the scales. I think I weighed ninety-nine pounds, I was almost five feet tall, so it couldn't have been *that* bad, but my name was high up in the alphabet and the continuing screams of delighted discovery more or less obscured the fact that there were at least two boys (one the pudgy red-headed kid) who weighed more than I did, to say nothing of that new foreign girl with the moustache, but she didn't count because she was only with us for about a month; I had to live in that town. So for the next two years, until I went to high school, I was the fattest kid in the class.

You may not be able to see it, but I still am.

I was marked, I suffered, I have carried that fat girl around with me for the rest of my life since then, and although I am a reasonable size ten she is still inside me, lurking just beneath the surface, crouched and ready to spring. I will weigh daily and learn to love the vegetable, I will walk miles or swim endlessly to keep her locked away.

For those of us who have been fat, ever, even as unwitting infants, there is the spectral presence of hundreds of thousands of fat cells lying in wait for just the right quart of ice cream or 24-inch pizza that will cause them to expand into rosy fullness, and as we grow older only constant vigilance and unremitting effort will keep them flattened. On the other hand, research indicates we may have some admirable qualities.

One school of psychologists holds that fat people may be fat not because they're starving every living minute but because of a heightened sensitivity. Surroundings, visual cues, pleasant smells can trigger eating, but the food has to be attractive. According to psychologist Stanley Schachter, fat freshmen eschewed the Columbia University dining hall precisely because the food and surroundings were unattractive. Should we condemn such a highly developed aesthetic sense? We admire other manifestations of this sensitivity: "visuals" who transform every room they occupy by careful placement of beloved objects; writers who can tell you every detail about a room they've just been in or render entire landscapes from memory; people who dress with style.

As a thin fat person grappling with all those fat cells, I find I collect paintings, catalogue every room I go into and dress to the eyeballs every chance I get; I would never make implications about any other writer, house freak or snappy dresser, but now that I manage to weigh one hundred and fifteen most of the time, I can't help but wonder whether the one has more than a little to do with the other. I keep my fat girl locked inside, but I can't despise her, because our relationship is too complex.

The terrible thing is that I never stop wondering what she looks like, and I have to keep a firm grip on the hand that holds the fork because the temptation is to let her loose and find out. One of the characters in Somerset Maugham's "Three Fat Women of Antibes" says, wistfully, "I haven't eaten potatoes for twenty-five years." I know just how she feels. A beautifully slender friend of mine, who is now in her sixties, says, "I'm hungry all the time." I know what she means, too. I'm getting there. Is it worth it?

Oh hell, what if I just let go? Although nobody can predict the ravages of age or weakened will, the chances are I'll never do it. In the seventh grade, I was the fattest kid in the class, and I never got over it. I remember the guilt over each sundae, the self-hatred, the resolution and inevitable fall; I remember kindly relatives saying, "Oh, well, it's your birthday," or "Well, you are on vacation," or, "After all, I made your favorite kind of pie," adding, in an indulgent aside, "Baby fat; she'll outgrow it." I remember them turning on me in the next second in what was to me a totally incomprehensible reversal, saying, "You really are going to have to do something about yourself." I remember putting my faith in vertical stripes and baggy sweaters designed to cover a multitude of sins behind, avoiding three-way mirrors and trying to find fatter people to stand next to so I wouldn't look so bad; I remember *knowing*, and I will resort to whatever extremes of self-denial I have to—anything to keep from going that way again.

It is an increasing consolation to discover that I am not alone. There are those of us who carry shadows of former, fatter selves, and we have been joined by an even greater number of victims of time and age and circumstance. The bitter truth is that it doesn't matter how thin you are in your teens or early twenties; unless you are an anomaly, your body needs fewer calories for every year it ages after twenty-six. After a certain age, even the most lissome person is liable to have to work to stay that way. For some the reckoning doesn't come until thirty-five, or even fifty, but it comes at last. Most of those skinny kids who laughed at me in the seventh grade are on perpetual diets now—or else they have gotten fat . . .

There are bound to be a few gorgeous exceptions who love food and can eat anything they want and I hate them, but usually when I pursue a certain morbid habit of mine and ask a skinny what he eats, he's likely to say he happens not to *like* desserts, or starches, or second helpings, or any of those wonderful excesses most of us don't dare allow but can't stop thinking about. (In "The Ordeal of Fats Goldberg," Calvin Trillin asks the now skinny Fats how he feels about his life of self-denial. "There is a lot of pain involved," says Fats. "A lot of pain. I can't stress that enough.") Genuine skinnies don't care what they eat or whether they eat. So much for them. I could never trust a man who eats less than I do.

For the rest of us, there is the consolation of a sort of grim camaraderie. We enjoy what we eat, we love it and we miss it. We may eat for pleasure or for extra energy or consolation in time of stress or because there is something special about sharing good food with good friends, but never only for fuel and always caring about what it is we eat or do not eat, and for the most part, we are almost always on a diet.

All the slimming, swimming, exercise and self-denial are done with a double aim in mind. One is the reasonable waistline: nobody is going to call *me* the fattest kid in the class. The other is that wonderful moment when it's OK to chuck it all and have the tacos *and* the cheese enchiladas, or go ahead and *eat* that Napoleon, always with the idea that this is a fling and it's back to short rations tomorrow. We tell ourselves there is something to be said for judicious eating: when they come, the rich moments mean so much more.

The horrible truth is, in most cases, this isn't a matter of getting any thinner. It's strictly a maintenance operation, the regimen necessary to keep from getting fat. A terrible way to live.

One party drunk became enraged at the very idea, saying he thought it was obscene for a person to keep gaining the same two pounds every weekend and dropping them every week. OK, fella, what if we just kept on gaining and never lost?

It seems logical to wonder how the other half lives.

The axiom goes: everybody loves a fat man, but does everybody, really?

Despite organizations formed to trumpet the opposite, we don't, really. Watching fat people at the buffet table or the soda fountain, we note the heaping plates or the extra whipped cream and think: uh-*huh*. With a few clandestine calories under our belts, we say we understand; we sympathize, we empathize, but at the same time we are telling them they look just fine to *us*, there is an undercurrent of righteousness which betrays our dazzling incomprehension: Listen, nobody has to be that fat. All it takes is a little exercise and a steady hand on the refrigerator door.

Anybody who has ever dieted knows that dieters will talk about food the way jailbirds must talk about sex. In a strange, vicarious way, this fascination of ours extends to people who are fat. We watch them with curiosity; we read about them. Starving, we try to envision their orgies; we read the reducing ads, enthralled. When we have the opportunity (only after casting shifty looks about to see that none of *them* are listening) we swap stories. There was the girl at Vassar who would lock herself in her room with sixty dollars' worth of groceries and emerge some days later, giddy and sated. There was Jean Stafford's girlhood friend, who denied all knowledge of the empty five-pound chocolate pudding tin she had hidden under the sofa. "The dog must have gotten it," she said, and nobody had the heart to ask her how the dog had managed the key to open the tin. Her roommates also forebore asking her how the half-eaten stick of butter found its way into her underwear drawer. Somebody else knew a girl who begged her roommate to keep her on a diet and then roused herself every morning at four o'clock so she could gorge on Hershey bars before the sun came up. One bunch of desperate dieters in Hollywood formed a chapter of Fooda-holics Anonymous, which involved frantic middle-of-the-night phone calls: "Listen, Harry, I've just made a whole spaghetti dinner with antipasto and a chocolate cake and I'm here all by myself and I'm scared of what I'm going to do." "Hold tight, sweetie, flush it all down the toilet and I'll be right over to talk you through." There was the Fattest Man in the World, named Robert Hughes. According to the *Guinness Book of World Records,* he weighed 1,096 pounds at the height of his career and was so big he had to be buried in a piano case. There was Mr. Thrale, who, it is rumored, ate himself to death, and there was William Howard Taft . . .

I have to admit that as a fat child, I turned to the confessions in the women's magazines for consolation. Look, here was a lady who weighed *three hundred pounds* until she took herself in hand. Here's a picture of her at a hundred and fifty; gee, next to her I don't look so bad. Look, here it tells you how to do it: the ads. Every ad followed a predictable pattern: I was *so* fat that——Enthralling stuff. Then there were the comics, the pop songs, including "Huggin' and a' Chalkin'," "The Too Fat Polka" and "Mr. Five by Five." Reading, listening, I could laugh and point a finger: "Hoo boy, FAT," hearing at the same time the inner voice: *I know just how it feels.*

When I grew up to be a writer, I found I had at least two "fat" stories in me, and perhaps because I was alert to the subject, I discovered that a number of other writers were interested in fat: hyperbolic physical description, the pathology of compulsive eating, the mystery of size. I think I can account for my own interest; it may go back as far as the first dread day in grammar school; when I write about fat, or compulsive eating, I may only be in doubt, casting that first stone. *Hey look, it isn't me,* or: *Maybe it's you.*

The extraordinary thing is that dozens of other writers seem to share my fascination. Once I had discovered "The Three Fat Women of Antibes" and Jean Stafford's "The Echo and the Nemesis," I thought there might be enough written to fill a fat book. Instead I found enough to fill wheelbarrows. Everybody I talked to had suggestions; everybody seemed to know fat, or, the other side of the coin, staying thin.

Although fat people often pretend to be jolly and we pretend to laugh at them, we know that fat isn't funny, and so do they. Fat captures the imagination, inspiring painters and writers; it troubles doctors and other researchers, who spend entire lifetimes trying to explore the causes.

Fat people are our monuments, our totems; they are emblems of much more complicated matters. They have a dignity of presence which commands our attention, although we cannot seem to agree what made them the way they are, or what they mean to us. Are they walking symbols of pain, or of want, or of appetite completely satisfied? If we laugh at them, it is an attempt, literally, to bring them down to size.

Writing, we may make up stories about how good-natured they are, or how vicious ("The Echo and the Nemesis," by Jean Stafford). We may create cadenzas on their menus (John Deck's "Notes: What I Think Pudding Says") or glorify their debauchery (Burr Snider's "Fat City"). We investigate and write with a fervor verging on prurience. Look at them. Why do they draw our eyes even when we are pretending not to look? What makes them this way?

We wonder whether they are fat because of an extraordinary weakness or extraordinary want. Most fiction about fat people seems to center on the idea of love, or loss of love. In fiction about fat, food is never simply food. Although the authors' uses vary, food always stands for something more.

The ad men tell us, "Nothin' says lovin' like something from the oven." Some psychiatrists say food equals love equals sex, but we have to wonder: Is that instead of love, or sex, or is it besides? Doctors differ. Laymen wonder: Hey, how far do these prodigious appetites extend? Do they extend all the way across the board, or has the appetite for the one stifled and replaced the appetite for the other? It *is* meals, isn't it? It's meals all the way down: legs of lamb and loaves of bread and entire apple pies. It's not what they did, it's what they ate ("The Food Farm"), right?

Not necessarily. In an abstract by psychologists Ronald A. Schwartz, David B. Hershenson and William G. Shipman of Dr. Schwartz's dissertation on the sexual behavior of obese women, the psychologists discovered that fat wives' sexual appetites seemed livelier than those of thin subjects.

They wrote, "One of the prevailing hypotheses concerning the etiology of obesity focuses on love deprivation as the root of the problem. Some people reared without affection turn to food as a substitute for love. In the totality of the sexual act—the bodily contact, the attendant expressions of endearment, the mutual giving—the obese woman probably derives relief from this emotional hunger. The desire for coitus is simply one expression of a more general desire to obtain the affection of which she was deprived as a child; overnutrition is another."

Dr. Shipman has arrived at an interesting ramification of this theory. Looking over the data, he discovered that these obese wives were dominant personalities, married to dominant and successful men, which he suspects leads to power struggles in the marriage bed. When the women are disappointed, they may make up the difference with food. He writes, "My experience suggests a different motto than yours. I find that inside every fat person is a thin, bad one that they are desperately trying not to let out."

There are almost as many theories as there are inves-
tigators. Some believe in love deprivation as the trigger,
others in acute visual and tactile sensitivity, others in
physical differences and even laziness which may be either
a cause or a symptom. The rest of us, skinny fat people and
parlor psychologists all, have our own theories and expand
on them, but what do we know after all?

Fat—gross, monumental fatness—remains fascinating
because it remains a mystery. The patterns seem familiar:
depression and hunger, guilt and self-reproach, expectation and disappointment, all common currency to anyone
who has ever known an alcoholic—or been on a diet. We
see ourselves in them yet we do not see ourselves exactly;
we too have had the ice cream parlor orgies, the pasta
festivals, the starchy excesses and midnight regrets—but
we have stopped, retrenched, rearranged ourselves. They
have not. What makes the difference?

Perhaps because we'll never know, we continue to describe and embroider and investigate and theorize. Or
maybe the tales we swap, or write, carry a certain aura of
confession. It may be that some of us are in a class with
members of AA, or the Weight Watchers, who stand up in
front of one another to exchange tales of dietary debauchery simply to gain the strength to go on. There is a certain
voyeurism involved, but there is something more.

I think we are a little afraid, partly for them, partly for
ourselves. Although we are not them, we are enough *like*
them to be frightened. We jog or swim and starve and
continue to spin stories and bore each other with diet tips
like travelers gathered around a fire trying to ward off the
dreadful night.

All right. When I'm on a diet, which is usually five and
a half days out of seven, I don't eat anything white. No
potatoes, no bread, no ice cream or cake. Starch is death.

But listen, everybody. Yesterday was a really bad day, so
at three P.M. I went down to the kitchen and made a pot of
fudge and ate it all myself.

Perhaps at the back of all our minds there sits the same huge, solitary figure, unassuagable, eating and weeping.

— *Kit Reed*

THE THREE FAT WOMEN OF ANTIBES

by *W. Somerset Maugham*

ONE was called Mrs. Richman and she was a widow. The second was called Mrs. Sutcliffe; she was American and she had divorced two husbands. The third was called Miss Hickson and she was a spinster. They were all in the comfortable forties and they were all well off. Mrs. Sutcliffe had the odd first name of Arrow. When she was young and slender she had liked it well enough. It suited her and the jests it occasioned though too often repeated were very flattering; she was not disinclined to believe that it suited her character too: it suggested directness, speed and purpose. She liked it less now that her delicate features had grown muzzy with fat, that her arms and shoulders were so substantial and her hips so massive. It was increasingly difficult to find dresses to make her look as she liked to look. The jests her name gave rise to now were made behind her back and she very well knew that they were far from obliging. But she was by no means resigned to middle age. She still wore blue to bring out the colour of her eyes and, with the help of art, her fair hair had kept its lustre. What she liked about Beatrice Richman and Frances Hickson was that they were both so much fatter than she, it made her look quite slim; they were both of them older and much inclined to treat her as a little young thing. It was not disagreeable. They were good-natured women and they chaffed her pleasantly about her beaux; they had both given up the thought of that kind of nonsense, indeed Miss Hickson had never given it a moment's consideration, but they were sympathetic to her flirtations. It was understood that one of these days Arrow would make a third man happy.

"Only you mustn't get any heavier, darling," said Mrs. Richman.

"And for goodness' sake make certain of his bridge," said Miss Hickson.

They saw for her a man of about fifty, but well-preserved and of distinguished carriage, an admiral on the retired list and a good golfer, or a widower without encumbrances, but in any case with a substantial income. Arrow listened to them amiably, and kept to herself that fact that this was not at all her idea. It was true that she would have liked to marry again, but her fancy turned to a dark slim Italian with flashing eyes and a sonorous title or to a Spanish don of noble lineage; and not a day more than thirty. There were times when, looking at herself in her mirror, she was certain she did not look any more than that herself.

They were great friends, Miss Hickson, Mrs. Richman and Arrow Sutcliffe. It was their fat that had brought them together and bridge that had cemented their alliance. They had met first at Carlsbad, where they were staying at the same hotel and were treated by the same doctor who used them with the same ruthlessness. Beatrice Richman was enormous. She was a handsome woman, with fine eyes, rouged cheeks and painted lips. She was very well content to be a widow with a handsome fortune. She adored her food. She liked bread and butter, cream, potatoes and suet puddings, and for eleven months of the year ate pretty well everything she had a mind to, and for one month went to Carlsbad to reduce. But every year she grew fatter. She upbraided the doctor, but got no sympathy from him. He pointed out to her various plain and simple facts.

"But if I'm never to eat a thing I like, life isn't worth living," she expostulated.

He shrugged his disapproving shoulders. Afterwards she told Miss Hickson that she was beginning to suspect he wasn't so clever as she had thought. Miss Hickson gave a great guffaw. She was that sort of woman. She had a deep bass voice, a large flat sallow face from which twinkled little bright eyes; she walked with a slouch, her hands in her pockets, and when she could do so without exciting attention smoked a long cigar. She dressed as like a man as she could.

"What the deuce should I look like in frills and furbelows?" she said. "When you're as fat as I am you may just as well be comfortable."

She wore tweeds and heavy boots and whenever she could went about bareheaded. But she was as strong as an ox and boasted that few men could drive a longer ball than she. She was plain of speech, and she could swear more variously than a stevedore. Though her name was Frances she preferred to be called Frank. Masterful, but with tact, it was her jovial strength of character that held the three together. They drank their waters together, had their baths at the same hour, they took their strenuous walks together, pounded about the tennis court with a professional to make them run, and ate at the same table their sparse and regulated meals. Nothing impaired their good humour but the scales, and when one or other of them weighed as much on one day as she had the day before neither Frank's coarse jokes, the *bonhomie* of Beatrice nor Arrow's pretty kittenish ways sufficed to dispel the gloom. Then drastic measures were resorted to, the culprit went to bed for twenty-four hours and nothing passed her lips but the doctor's famous vegetable soup which tasted like hot water in which a cabbage had been well rinsed.

Never were three women greater friends. They would have been independent of anyone else if they had not needed a fourth at bridge. They were fierce, enthusiastic players and the moment the day's cure was over they sat down at the bridge table. Arrow, feminine as she was, played the best game of the three, a hard, brilliant game, in which she showed no mercy and never conceded a point or failed to take advantage of a mistake. Beatrice was solid and reliable. Frank was dashing; she was a great theorist, and had all the authorities at the tip of her tongue. They had long arguments over the rival systems. They bombarded one another with Culbertson and Sims. It was obvious that not one of them ever played a card without fifteen good reasons, but it was also obvious from the subsequent conversation that there were fifteen equally good reasons why she should not have played it. Life would have been perfect, even with the prospect of twenty-four hours of that filthy soup when the doctor's rotten (Beatrice) bloody (Frank) lousy (Arrow) scales pretended one hadn't lost an ounce in two days, if only there had not been this constant difficulty of finding someone to play with them who was in their class.

It was for this reason that on the occasion with which this narrative deals Frank invited Lena Finch to come and stay with them at Antibes. They were spending some weeks there on Frank's suggestion. It seemed absurd to her, with her common sense, that immediately the cure was over Beatrice who always lost twenty pounds should by giving way to her ungovernable appetite put it all on again. Beatrice was weak. She needed a person of strong will to watch her diet. She proposed then that on leaving Carlsbad they should take a house at Antibes, where they could get plenty of exercise—everyone knew that nothing slimmed you like swimming—and as far as possible could go on with the cure. With a cook of their own they could at least avoid things that were obviously fattening. There was no reason why they should not all lose several pounds more. It seemed a very good idea. Beatrice knew what was good for her, and she could resist temptation well enough if temptation was not put right under her nose. Besides, she liked gambling, and a flutter at the Casino two or three times a week would pass the time very pleasantly. Arrow adored Antibes, and she would be looking her best after a month at Carlsbad. She could just pick and choose among the young Italians, the passionate Spaniards, the gallant Frenchmen, and the long-limbed English who sauntered about all day in bathing trunks and gay-coloured dressing-gowns. The plan worked very well. They had a grand time.

Two days a week they ate nothing but hard-boiled eggs and raw tomatoes and they mounted the scales every morning with light hearts. Arrow got down to eleven stone and felt just like a girl; Beatrice and Frank by standing in a certain way just avoided the thirteen. The machine they had bought registered kilogrameś, and they got extraordinarily clever at translating these in the twinkling of an eye to pounds and ounces.

But the fourth at bridge continued to be the difficulty. This person played like a foot, the other was so slow that it drove you frantic, one was quarrelsome, another was a bad loser, a third was next door to a crook. It was strange how hard it was to find exactly the player you wanted.

One morning when they were sitting in pyjamas on the terrace overlooking the sea, drinking their tea (without milk or sugar) and eating a rusk prepared by Dr. Hudebert and guaranteed not to be fattening, Frank looked up from her letters.

"Lena Finch is coming down to the Riviera," she said.

"Who's she?" asked Arrow.

"She married a cousin of mine. He died a couple of months ago and she's just recovering from a nervous breakdown. What about asking her to come here for a fortnight?"

"Does she play bridge?" asked Beatrice.

"You bet your life she does," boomed Frank in her deep voice. "And a damned good game too. We should be absolutely independent of outsiders."

"How old is she?" asked Arrow.

"Same age as I am."

"That sounds all right."

It was settled. Frank, with her usual decisiveness, stalked out as soon as she had finished her breakfast to send a wire, and three days later Lena Finch arrived. Frank met her at the station. She was in deep but not obtrusive mourning for the recent death of her husband. Frank had not seen her for two years. She kissed her warmly and took a good look at her.

"You're very thin, darling," she said.

Lena smiled bravely.

"I've been through a good deal lately. I've lost a lot of weight."

Frank sighed, but whether from sympathy with her cousin's sad loss, or from envy, was not obvious.

Lena was not, however, unduly depressed, and after a quick bath was quite ready to accompany Frank to Eden Roc. Frank introduced the stranger to her two friends and they sat down in what was known as the Monkey House. It was an enclosure covered with glass overlooking the sea, with a bar at the back, and it was crowded with chattering people in bathing costumes, pyjamas or dressing-gowns, who were seated at the tables having drinks. Beatrice's soft heart went out to the lorn widow, and Arrow, seeing that she was pale, quite ordinary to look at and probably forty-eight, was prepared to like her very much. A waiter approached them.

"What will you have, Lena dear?" Frank asked.

"Oh, I don't know, what you all have, a dry Martini or a White Lady."

Arrow and Beatrice gave her a quick look. Everyone knows how fattening cocktails are.

"I daresay you're tired after your journey," said Frank kindly.

She ordered a dry Martini for Lena and a mixed lemon and orange juice for herself and her two friends.

"We find alcohol isn't very good in all this heat," she explained.

"Oh, it never affects me at all," Lena answered airily. "I like cocktails."

Arrow went very slightly pale under her rouge (neither she nor Beatrice ever wet their faces when they bathed and they thought it absurd of Frank, a woman of her size, to pretend she liked diving) but she said nothing. The conversation was gay and easy, they all said the obvious things with gusto, and presently they strolled back to the villa for luncheon.

In each napkin were two little antifat rusks. Lena gave a bright smile as she put them by the side of her plate.

"May I have some bread?" she asked.

The grossest indecency would not have fallen on the ears of those three women with such a shock. Not one of them had eaten bread for ten years. Even Beatrice, greedy as she was, drew the line there. Frank, the good hostess, recovered herself first.

"Of course, darling," she said and turning to the butler asked him to bring some.

"And some butter," said Lena in that pleasant easy way of hers.

There was a moment's embarrassed silence.

"I don't know if there's any in the house," said Frank, "but I'll enquire. There may be some in the kitchen."

"I adore bread and butter, don't you?" said Lena, turning to Beatrice.

Beatrice gave a sickly smile and an evasive reply. The butler brought a long crisp roll of French bread. Lena slit it in two and plastered it with the butter which was miraculously produced. A grilled sole was served.

"We eat very simply here," said Frank. "I hope you won't mind."

"Oh, no, I like my food very plain," said Lena as she took some butter and spread it over her fish. "As long as I can have bread and butter and potatoes and cream I'm quite happy."

The three friends exchanged a glance. Frank's great sallow face sagged a little and she looked with distaste at the dry, insipid sole on her plate. Beatrice came to the rescue.

"It's such a bore, we can't get cream here," she said. "It's one of the things one has to do without on the Riviera."

"What a pity," said Lena.

The rest of the luncheon consisted of lamb cutlets, with the fat carefully removed so that Beatrice should not be led astray, and spinach boiled in water, with stewed pears to end up with. Lena tasted her pears and gave the butler a look of enquiry. That resourceful man understood her at once and though powdered sugar had never been served at that table before handed her without a moment's hesitation a bowl of it. She helped herself liberally. The other three pretended not to notice. Coffee was served and Lena took three lumps of sugar in hers.

"You have a very sweet tooth," said Arrow in a tone which she struggled to keep friendly.

"We think saccharine so much more sweetening," said Frank, as she put a tiny tablet of it into her coffee.

"Disgusting stuff," said Lena.

Beatrice's mouth drooped at the corners, and she gave the lump sugar a yearning look.

"Beatrice," boomed Frank sternly.

Beatrice stifled a sigh, and reached for the saccharine.

Frank was relieved when they could sit down to the bridge table. It was plain to her that Arrow and Beatrice were upset. She wanted them to like Lena and she was anxious that Lena should enjoy her fortnight with them. For the first rubber Arrow cut with the newcomer.

"Do you play Vanderbilt or Culbertson?" she asked her.

"I have no conventions," Lena answered in a happy-go-lucky way, "I play by the light of nature."

"I play strict Culbertson," said Arrow acidly.

The three fat women braced themselves to the fray. No conventions indeed! They'd learn her. When it came to bridge even Frank's family feeling was forgotten and she settled down with the same determination as the others to trim the stranger in their midst. But the light of nature served Lena very well. She had a natural gift for the game and great experience. She played with imagination, quickly, boldly, and with assurance. The other players were in too high a class not to realise very soon that Lena knew what she was about, and since they were all thoroughly good-natured, generous women, they were gradually mollified. This was real bridge. They all enjoyed themselves. Arrow and Beatrice began to feel more kindly towards Lena, and

Frank, noticing this, heaved a fat sigh of relief. It was going to be a success.

After a couple of hours they parted, Frank and Beatrice to have a round of golf, and Arrow to take a brisk walk with a young Prince Roccamare whose acquaintance she had lately made. He was very sweet and young and good-looking. Lena said she would rest.

They met again just before dinner.

"I hope you've been all right, Lena dear," said Frank. "I was rather conscience-stricken at leaving you with nothing to do all this time."

"Oh, don't apologise. I had a lovely sleep and then I went down to Juan and had a cocktail. And d'you know what I discovered? You'll be so pleased. I found a dear little tea-shop where they've got the most beautiful thick fresh cream. I've ordered half a pint to be sent every day. I thought it would be my little contribution to the household."

Her eyes were shining. She was evidently expecting them to be delighted.

"How very kind of you," said Frank, with a look that sought to quell the indignation that she saw on the faces of her two friends. "But we never eat cream. In this climate it makes one so bilious."

"I shall have to eat it all myself then," said Lena cheerfully.

"Don't you ever think of your figure?" Arrow asked with icy deliberation.

"The doctor said I must eat."

"Did he say you must eat bread and butter and potatoes and cream?"

"Yes. That's what I thought you meant when you said you had simple food."

"You'll get simply enormous," said Beatrice.

Lena laughed gaily.

"No, I shan't. You see, nothing ever makes me fat. I've always eaten everything I wanted to and it's never had the slightest effect on me."

The stony silence that followed this speech was only broken by the entrance of the butler.

"Mademoiselle est servie," he announced.

They talked the matter over late that night, in Frank's room, after Lena had gone to bed. During the evening they had been furiously cheerful, and they had chaffed one another with a friendliness that would have taken in the keenest observer. But now they dropped the mask. Beatrice was sullen, Arrow was spiteful and Frank was unmanned.

"It's not very nice for me to sit there and see her eat all the things I particularly like," said Beatrice plaintively.

"It's not very nice for any of us," Frank snapped back.

"You should never have asked her here," said Arrow.

"How was I to know?" cried Frank.

"I can't help thinking that if she really cared for her husband she would hardly eat so much," said Beatrice. "He's only been buried two months. I mean, I think you ought to show some respect for the dead."

"Why can't she eat the same as we do?" asked Arrow viciously. "She's a guest."

"Well, you heard what she said. The doctor told her she must eat."

"Then she ought to go to a sanatorium."

"It's more than flesh and blood can stand, Frank," moaned Beatrice.

"If I can stand it you can stand it."

"She's your cousin, she's not our cousin," said Arrow. "I'm not going to sit there for fourteen days and watch that woman make a hog of herself."

"It's so vulgar to attach all this importance to food," Frank boomed, and her voice was deeper than ever. "After all the only thing that counts really is spirit."

"Are you calling *me* vulgar, Frank?" asked Arrow with flashing eyes.

"No, of course she isn't," interrupted Beatrice.

"I wouldn't put it past you to go down in the kitchen when we're all in bed and have a good square meal on the sly."

Frank sprang to her feet.

"How dare you say that, Arrow! I'd never ask anybody to do what I'm not prepared to do myself. Have you known me all these years and do you think me capable of such a mean thing?"

"How is it you never take off any weight then?"

Frank gave a gasp and burst into a flood of tears.

"What a cruel thing to say! I've lost pounds and pounds."

She wept like a child. Her vast body shook and great tears splashed on her mountainous bosom.

"Darling, I didn't mean it," cried Arrow.

She threw herself on her knees and enveloped what she could of Frank in her own plump arms. She wept and the mascara ran down her cheeks.

"D'you mean to say I don't look thinner?" Frank sobbed. "After all I've gone through."

"Yes, dear, of course you do," cried Arrow through her tears. "Everybody's noticed it."

Beatrice, though naturally of a placid disposition, began to cry gently. It was very pathetic. Indeed, it would have been a hard heart that failed to be moved by the sight of Frank, that lion-hearted woman, crying her eyes out. Presently, however, they dried their tears and had a little brandy and water, which every doctor had told them was the least fattening thing they could drink, and then they felt much better. They decided that Lena should have the nourishing food that had been ordered her and they made a solemn resolution not to let it disturb their equanimity. She was certainly a first-rate bridge player and after all it was only for a fortnight. They would do whatever they could to make her stay enjoyable. They kissed one another warmly and separated for the night feeling strangely uplifted. Nothing should interfere with the wonderful friendship that had brought so much happiness into their three lives.

But human nature is weak. You must not ask too much of it. They ate grilled fish while Lena ate macaroni sizzling

with cheese and butter; they ate grilled cutlets and boiled
spinach while Lena ate *pâté de foie gras;* twice a week they
ate hard-boiled eggs and raw tomatoes, while Lena ate peas
swimming in cream and potatoes cooked in all sorts of
delicious ways. The chef was a good chef and he leapt at
the opportunity afforded him to send up one dish more
rich, tasty and succulent than the other.

"Poor Jim," sighed Lena, thinking of her husband, "he
loved French cooking."

The butler disclosed the fact that he could make half a
dozen kinds of cocktail and Lena informed them that the
doctor had recommended her to drink burgundy at luncheon and champagne at dinner. The three fat women per-
severed. They were gay, chatty and even hilarious (such is
the natural gift that women have for deception) but Beatrice grew limp and forlorn, and Arrow's tender blue eyes
acquired a steely glint. Frank's deep voice grew more rau-
cous. It was when they played bridge that the strain showed
itself. They had always been fond of talking over their
hands, but their discussions had been friendly. Now a distinct bitterness crept in and sometimes one pointed out a
mistake to another with quite unnecessary frankness. Discussion turned to argument and argument to altercation.
Sometimes the session ended in angry silence. Once Frank
accused Arrow of deliberately letting her down. Two or
three times Beatrice, the softest of the three, was reduced
to tears. On another occasion Arrow flung down her cards
and swept out of the room in a pet. Their tempers were
getting frayed. Lena was the peacemaker.

"I think it's such a pity to quarrel over bridge," she said.
"After all, it's only a game."

It was all very well for her. She had had a square meal
and half a bottle of champagne. Besides, she had phe-
nomenal luck. She was winning all their money. The score
was put down in a book after each session, and hers
mounted up day after day with unfailing regularity. Was
there no justice in the world? They began to hate one
another. And though they hated her too they could not

resist confiding in her. Each of them went to her separately and told her how detestable the others were. Arrow said she was sure it was bad for her to see so much of women so much older than herself. She had a good mind to sacrifice her share of the lease and go to Venice for the rest of the summer. Frank told Lena that with her masculine mind it was too much to expect that she could be satisfied with anyone so frivolous as Arrow and so frankly stupid as Beatrice.

"I must have intellectual conversation," she boomed. "When you have a brain like mine you've got to consort with your intellectual equals."

Beatrice only wanted peace and quiet.

"Really I hate women," she said. "They're so unreliable; they're so malicious."

By the time Lena's fortnight drew to its close the three fat women were barely on speaking terms. They kept up appearances before Lena, but when she was not there made no pretences. They had got past quarrelling. They ignored one another, and when this was not possible treated each other with icy politeness.

Lena was going to stay with friends on the Italian Riviera and Frank saw her off by the same train as that by which she had arrived. She was taking away with her a lot of their money.

"I don't know how to thank you," she said, as she got into the carriage. "I've had a wonderful visit."

If there was one thing that Frank Hickson prided herself on more than on being a match for any man it was that she was a gentlewoman, and her reply was perfect in its combination of majesty and graciousness.

"We've all enjoyed having you here, Lena," she said. "It's been a real treat."

But when she turned away from the departing train she heaved such a vast sigh of relief that the platform shook beneath her. She flung back her massive shoulders and strode home to the villa.

"Ouf!" she roared at intervals. "Ouf!"

She changed into her one-piece bathing-suit, put on her espadrilles and a man's dressing-gown (no nonsense about it) and went to Eden Roc. There was still time for a bathe before luncheon. She passed through the Monkey House, looking about her to say good morning to anyone she knew, for she felt on a sudden at peace with mankind, and then stopped dead still. She could not believe her eyes. Beatrice was sitting at one of the tables, by herself; she wore the pyjamas she had bought at Molyneux's a day or two before, she had a string of pearls round her neck, and Frank's quick eyes saw that she had just had her hair waved; her cheeks, her eyes, her lips were made up. Fat, nay vast, as she was, none could deny that she was an extremely handsome woman. But what was she doing? With the slouching gait of the Neanderthal man which was Frank's characteristic walk she went up to Beatrice. In her black bathing-dress Frank looked like the huge cetacean which the Japanese catch in the Torres Straits and which the vulgar call a sea-cow.

"Beatrice, what are you doing?" she cried in her deep voice.

It was like the roll of thunder in the distant mountains. Beatrice looked at her coolly.

"Eating," she answered.

"Damn it, I can see you're eating."

In front of Beatrice was a plate of *croissants* and a plate of butter, a pot of strawberry jam, coffee and a jug of cream. Beatrice was spreading butter thick on the delicious hot bread, covering this with jam, and then pouring the thick cream over all.

"You'll kill yourself," said Frank.

"I don't care," mumbled Beatrice with her mouth full.

"You'll put on pounds and pounds."

"Go to hell!"

She actually laughed in Frank's face. My God, how good those *croissants* smelt!

"I'm disappointed in you, Beatrice. I thought you had more character."

"It's your fault. That blasted woman. You would have her down. For a fortnight I've watched her gorge like a hog. It's more than flesh and blood can stand. I'm going to have one square meal if I bust."

The tears welled up to Frank's eyes. Suddenly she felt very weak and womanly. She would have liked a strong man to take her on his knee and pet her and cuddle her and call her little baby names. Speechless she sank down on a chair by Beatrice's side. A waiter came up. With a pathetic gesture she waved towards the coffee and *croissants.*

"I'll have the same," she sighed.

She listlessly reached out her hand to take a roll, but Beatrice snatched away the plate.

"No, you don't," she said. "You wait till you get your own."

Frank called her a name which ladies seldom apply to one another in affection. In a moment the waiter brought her *croissants,* butter, jam and coffee.

"Where's the cream, you fool?" she roared like a lioness at bay.

She began to eat. She ate gluttonously. The place was beginning to fill up with bathers coming to enjoy a cocktail or two after having done their duty by the sun and the sea. Presently Arrow strolled along with Prince Roccamare. She had on a beautiful silk wrap which she held tightly round her with one hand in order to look as slim as possible and she bore her head high so that he should not see her double chin. She was laughing gaily. She felt like a girl. He had just told her (in Italian) that her eyes made the blue of the Mediterranean look like pea-soup. He left her to go into the men's room to brush his sleek black hair and they arranged to meet in five minutes for a drink. Arrow walked on to the women's room to put a little more rouge on her cheeks and a little more red on her lips. On her way she caught sight of Frank and Beatrice. She stopped. She could hardly believe her eyes.

"My God!" she cried. "You beasts. You hogs." She seized a chair. "Waiter."

Her appointment went clean out of her head. In the twinkling of an eye the waiter was at her side.

"Bring me what these ladies are having," she ordered.

Frank lifted her great heavy head from her plate.

"Bring me some *pâté de foie gras,*" she boomed.

"Frank!" cried Beatrice.

"Shut up."

"All right. I'll have some too."

The coffee was brought and the hot rolls and cream and the *pâté de foie gras* and they set to. They spread the cream on the *pâté* and they ate it. They devoured great spoonfuls of jam. They crunched the delicious crisp bread voluptuously. What was love to Arrow then? Let the Prince keep his palace in Rome and his castle in the Apennines. They did not speak. What they were about was much too serious. They ate with solemn, ecstatic fervour.

"I haven't eaten potatoes for twenty-five years," said Frank in a far-off brooding tone.

"Waiter," cried Beatrice, "bring fried potatoes for three."

"Très bien, Madame."

The potatoes were brought. Not all the perfumes of Arabia smelt so sweet. They ate them with their fingers.

"Bring me a dry Martini," said Arrow.

"You can't have a dry Martini in the middle of a meal, Arrow," said Frank.

"Can't I? You wait and see."

"All right then. Bring me a double dry Martini," said Frank.

"Bring three double dry Martinis," said Beatrice.

They were brought and drunk at a gulp. The women looked at one another and sighed. The misunderstandings of the last fortnight dissolved and the sincere affection each had for the other welled up again in their hearts. They could hardly believe that they had ever contemplated the possibility of severing a friendship that had brought them so much solid satisfaction. They finished the potatoes.

"I wonder if they've got any chocolate éclairs," said Beatrice.

"Of course they have."

And of course they had. Frank thrust one whole into her huge mouth, swallowed it and seized another, but before she ate it she looked at the other two and plunged a vindictive dagger into the heart of the monstrous Lena.

"You can say what you like, but the truth is she played a damned rotten game of bridge, really."

"Lousy," agreed Arrow.

But Beatrice suddenly thought she would like a meringue.

FAT MAN

by **George Garrett**

O flesh, my tyrant wife, my shrew,
old slattern, what's to become of you?
Of *us?* It's true I have to hate
the way you smirk from mirrors, float
in steaming tubs, sweat on summer days,
or, shameless, writhe in nets of eyes
that measure all your bulk and girth.
It's you I love although I curse your birth.

What is to love? To love's to dance.
The spirit leads the flesh. Without a wince
the flesh should follow and should smile.
A map of all of you shows miles
of frowns. I study you and weep
for pity's sake—the only crop I reap.
I'll never leave you, cruel and fair,
who leave me panting halfway up the stair.

Abraham's Knife and Other Poems, by George Garrett (Chapel Hill: The University of North Carolina Press).

THE ORDEAL OF FATS GOLDBERG

by *Calvin Trillin*

Larry Goldberg, the pizza baron, is slim, but I still think of him as Fats Goldberg. So does he. Although he has "been down," as he puts it, for twelve years, after twenty-five years of exceptional fatness, he sees himself not as a man who weighs one hundred and sixty pounds but as a man who is constantly in danger of weighing three hundred twenty. "Inside, I'm still a fat man," he sometimes says. When Fats and I were boys in Kansas City, he was already renowned for his corpulence—though I can't say I was ever approached about posing for Refugee Relief ads in those days myself. During college, when Fats weighed three hundred pounds and was known to some as Three Cases Goldberg, I occasionally saw him at the University of Missouri, where he was one of a number of storied eaters. According to one tale, when a restaurant near the campus instituted a policy of giving customers all they wanted to eat on Sunday nights for a dollar thirty-five, a fraternity brother of Fats' called Hog Silverman, who weighed less than two and a half cases, went over one Sunday night and put it out of business. Fats was known not only for that kind of single-sitting tour de force but for the fact that he never stopped eating. When he talks about those days, a lot of his sentences begin with phrases like "Then on the way to lunch I'd stop off at the Tastee-Freez . . ."

Fats says that he did not get fat on *coq au vin*. "In the quantities I was eating, nobody could have afforded gourmet food," he has said. "I'm one of the great all-time junk eaters." Candy bars. Lunch-meat sandwiches on white

"The Ordeal of Fats Goldberg," by Calvin Trillin, copyright © 1971, by Calvin Trillin. Originally appeared in *The New Yorker*.

bread. Sweet rolls. Hamburgers. Chili dogs. Pizza. Not Goldberg's pizza—just pizza. At Missouri, Fats often brightened up the late afternoon with something called a Boston Sundae, which is, to the extent that it is describable, a milkshake with a floating sundae on top—a floating chocolate sundae with bananas if Fats happened to be the customer. I don't mean to imply that Fats was undiscriminating. There are good chili dogs and bad chili dogs. The only food that Fats still finds almost literally irresistible is a double cheeseburger with everything but onions at Winstead's, a hamburger place in Kansas City, and I must say that our afflictions differ only in that I prefer the double hamburger with everything and grilled onions. For a number of years, Fats was in the habit of reading the latest diet book at Winstead's—holding the book in one hand and a double cheeseburger with everything but onions in the other.

I didn't see Fats for ten years after college, and when I finally did see him I didn't recognize him. It was a Sunday morning, and I was at Ratner's, on Second Avenue. I was having eggs scrambled with lox and onions, and I was glancing around constantly, as I tend to do in Ratner's, to see if some other table was being given a roll basket with more of my favorite kind of onion rolls than our roll basket had. Fats didn't even look familiar. In fact, if we hadn't had some intimate discussions since then about Winstead's hamburgers and Charlie Bryant's barbecued spareribs, I might even now suspect him of being an impostor. Fats later told me that on the morning of May 1, 1959, while employed as a three-hundred-and-twenty-pound salesman of newspaper advertising space in Chicago, he had decided to lose weight. Naturally, he had made similar decisions several dozen times in the past, and he still doesn't know why he was finally able to stop eating. He is certain that it was not fear for his health; several years before, his reaction to a serious warning by a doctor in Kansas City was to think about it over three Winstead's cheeseburgers, a fresh-lime Coke, and a Frosty Malt. (A Frosty Malt is a kind of cross between a milkshake and a glassful of chocolate ice cream—described on the Winstead's menu as "The Drink You Eat with a Spoon.") On May 1, 1959, Fats started losing weight. He didn't use pills or gimmick diets. "It was cold turkey," he says now, referring to the method rather than the food. "I suffered." In a year, Fats weighed one-ninety. Then, gradually, he went down to one-sixty. In other words, by the time I saw him at Ratner's the Fats I had known was half gone.

Fats was still selling advertising space then, but he wasn't happy in his work. For a while, he tried standup comedy, working with a girl in a partnership called Berkowitz and Goldberg—an act that apparently inspired audiences all over town to puzzled silence. A few years ago, he went into the pizza-parlor business. He was armed not only with the gimmick of having a Jewish pizza parlor but with the recipe for an excellent version of what the connoisseurs call a Chicago pizza—characterized by a thick, crispy, and particularly fattening crust. Naturally, Goldberg's Pizzeria was a success. Fats himself became so celebrated that he was able to publish a pizza book—a volume that may add little to the literature of food but seems at least to have provided a resting place for some old jokes from the Berkowitz and Goldberg days. (One chapter is called "The Goldberg Variations, or How to Make Johann Sebastian Roll Over on His Bach.") Fats now has two thriving pizza parlors and is looking for a spot to open a third.

Although Fats enjoys the trappings of a pizza barony, he realizes that his most notable accomplishment is not having created a successful business but having stayed thin. Among his pizza customers are some experts in obesity, and they have informed him that any fat man who remains slim for twelve years can safely consider himself a medical phenomenon. (Since both of Goldberg's pizzerias display poster-size pictures of Fats when he weighed three cases, the subject of fatness often comes up, particularly on Sunday nights, the traditional time for diet resolutions.) Fats has been told that specialists can always make fat people thin through a variety of hospital treatments—treatments that a layman would probably summarize as solitary confinement—but once released the fat people almost invariably become fat again. Someone who has gone without a relapse since 1959 is so rare that one researcher from the Rockefeller University asked Fats if he would mind donating some of his fat cells for analysis. Researchers at Rockefeller and at Mt. Sinai Hospital have found that fat people who were fat as children have not only larger fat cells but more of them—a permanent extra helping that may come about through being overfed in the first few years of life. When a chronically fat person loses weight, all his fat cells just shrink temporarily, remaining available for reexpansion—or, as someone who apparently enjoys taunting the fatties once put it, "screaming to be refilled." Fat-cell research has led to the depressing speculation that a person who was fat as a child faces horrifying pressure to become fat again and again—as well as to the equally depressing speculation that blame for yet another atrocity might be laid at the feet of the Jewish Mother. Fats is unenthusiastic about the Rockefeller people's method of studying his fat cells, which would amount to withdrawing a section of tissue from the part of the body in which it is most accessible (or, as Fats sees it, "having three nurses stick an eight-inch needle in my *tushe*"), but lately he has begun to say that he would be willing to coöperate. The more he thinks about the effort required for a fat man to stay thin, the more he thinks that he is extraordinary enough to be a boon to medical research.

A couple of weeks ago, I happened to see a thin psychologist I know named Stanley Schachter, who has done a lot of research at Columbia on obesity, and I asked him if it was scientifically sound to consider Fats Goldberg truly amazing. After I had described Fats' accomplishment, Schachter seemed filled with admiration. According to Schachter's research, staying thin would be even more difficult for a pizza baron than for a run-of-the-mill fatty. The research indicates that what causes fat people to eat is not the physical sensations that go along with an empty stomach but what Schachter calls "external cues"—the sight of candy in the candy dish or the smell of hamburgers frying or the information that it is dinnertime or, in the case of poor Fats, the constant presence of delicious, aromatic pizza.

In fact, Schachter believes that fat people are unable to recognize the physical sensation of hunger—so that they actually eat less than thin people if external cues are missing. When two Columbia doctors, Theodore Van Italie and Sami Hashim, removed virtually all external cues—they allowed people to eat all they wanted of an almost tasteless liquid, but nothing else—the thin people ate about the same number of calories per day that they had eaten of normal food but the fat people ate so little that one of them lost more than two hundred pounds in eight months. Schachter has found that among a group of college students with roughly the same habits of synagogue attendance the fat ones are more likely to fast on Yom Kippur than the normal-sized ones—and that their fasting is more likely to be helped if they stay in the synagogue, where there are few food cues. The normal-sized ones get hungry. Normal people given food in a laboratory will eat less if their stomachs are full or if they're frightened, but if a plate of crackers is put in front of a fat person who has just eaten or who has been led to believe he is about to receive some electric shocks, he is likely to clean the plate anyway—or, in Schachter's terms, to eat until he is out of cues. The crackers have to be decent crackers, of course; fat people tend not to be interested in food that doesn't taste good.

After listening to Schachter explain the peculiar eating habits of fat people for a while, it occurred to me that what he had really discovered was that fat people are smarter than other people. For instance, in an experiment to test the hypothesis that fat people are less willing to work for their food than ordinary people, he found that the appeal of a bowl of almonds to normal-sized people who were filling out some meaningless forms he had concocted (Schachter is a very devious researcher) was unaffected by whether or not the almonds had shells on them. But when fat people were given the same test, only one out of twenty ate almonds that had to be shelled and nineteen out of twenty ate almonds that were already shelled. That seemed to me a simple matter of intelligence. Who wants to spend his time shelling almonds? Testing the same hypothesis, Schachter and some of his students loitered around Chinese restaurants and found that fat Occidentals are much less likely to try chopsticks than thin Occidentals.

"But the fat people behave the way any normal intelligent person would behave, Stanley," I said when I heard about that discovery.

Schachter didn't say anything. Then I began to realize that a lot of the fat-people habits he had talked about applied to me. I have always thought that anyone who sacrifices stuffing power by using chopsticks in a Chinese restaurant must be demented. Although I may have talked about being hungry from the moment I learned to talk, I am still not sure precisely what physical feeling people have in mind when they describe hunger. The last piece of food I left on my plate—that was in the fall of 1958, as I remember—had a bug on it. Schachter's theories, I decided, must be incorrect.

I tried to prove it to myself the next time I saw Fats, by asking him a question in what I knew was a somewhat misleading way.

"Do you ever get hungry, Fats?" I asked.

"You bet your booties I do!" Fats said.

That would show Schachter, I thought. But a few days later, when I asked Fats for an example of a time when it was particularly hard for him to avoid eating, he said, "Tonight when I passed that pizza stand on Eighth Street that has that great frozen custard, it almost killed me." External cue.

My discussion with Fats about hunger began at the Gaiety Delicatessen on Lexington Avenue, where he goes every day for a kind of lunchtime breakfast. Having been terrified by Schachter, I ordered the tuna-fish-salad plate with double coleslaw, hold the potato salad, and a low-calorie cream soda. Fats ate two scrambled eggs, sausages, a bagel with cream cheese, and four cups of coffee with a total of eight packets of sugar. "A fat man's got to have something to look forward to," Fats said. "When I'm reading in bed late at night, I think about being able to have this bagel and cream cheese the next day." Fats' secret of weight control is an eating schedule of uncompromising rigidity. His Gaiety meal varies daily only in how the eggs are done. In the evening, he has either a steak or half a chicken, baked in the pizza oven. (He is always careful to cut the chicken in half before baking and to put the unneeded half back into the refrigerator. "You have to pre-plan," he says. "A fat man always cleans his plate.") On Sunday night, he permits himself a quarter of a small sausage pizza in place of the steak or chicken, but then he works at the ovens trying to sweat it off. On Monday, he cheats to the extent of some bread or maybe a piece of pie. The schedule is maintained only in New York. Kansas City remains a free zone for Fats. He says that in the earlier years of his thinness a week's trip to Kansas City to visit his family would mean gaining seventeen pounds. Now, showing some restraint, he manages to hold it down to ten pounds.

A few days after our meeting at the Gaiety, Fats dropped by my house. (It had been a difficult few days for me: An Italian street fair was being held so close to my house that I had been able to convince myself I could smell the patently irresistible smell of frying sausages night and day.) I mentioned to Fats that a doctor I knew had said that in order to gain even fourteen pounds a week in Kansas City it would be necessary for Fats to consume an additional seventy-two hundred calories a day—or the equivalent of fifteen or twenty Winstead's cheeseburgers.

Fats considered that for a while. He didn't seem shocked.

"Just what *did* you eat on a big day in Kansas City the week you gained seventeen pounds?" I asked. I prepared to make a list.

"Well, for breakfast I'd have two eggs, six biscuits with butter and jelly, half a quart of milk, six link sausages, six strips of bacon, and a couple of homemade cinnamon rolls," Fats said. "Then I'd hit MacLean's Bakery. They have a kind of fried cinnamon roll I love. Maybe I'd have two or three of them. Then, on the way downtown to have lunch with somebody, I might stop at Kresge's and have two chili dogs and couple of root beers. Ever had their chili dogs?"

I shook my head.

"Greasiest chili dogs in the world," Fats said. "I love 'em. Then I'd go to lunch. What I really like for lunch is something like a hot beef sandwich or a hot turkey sandwich. Open-faced, loaded with that flour gravy. With mashed potatoes. Then Dutch apple pie. Kansas City is big on Dutch apple pie. Here they call it apple crumb or something. Then, sometimes in the afternoon, I'd pick up a pie—just an ordinary nine-inch pie—and go to my friend Matt Flynn's house, and we'd cut the pie down the middle and put half in a bowl for each of us and then take a quart of ice cream and cut that down the middle and put it on top of the pie. We'd wash it down with Pepsi-Cola. Sometimes Matt couldn't finish his and I'd have to finish it for him. Then that would be it until I stopped at my sister's house. She's very big on crunchy peanut butter. She even has peanut butter and jelly already mixed. They didn't have that when I was a kid. Then for dinner we'd maybe go to Charlie Bryant's or one of the barbecues out on the highway. At the movies, I'd always have a bag of corn and a big Coke and knock off a Payday candy bar. Payday is still my favorite candy bar. They're hard to get here, but they have very big distribution in Kansas City. Then we'd always end up at Winstead's, of course. Two double cheeseburgers with everything but onions, a fresh-lime Coke, and a Frosty Malt. If it was before eleven, I'd stop at the Zarda Dairy for one of their forty-nine-cent banana splits. Then when I'd get home maybe some cherry pie and a sixteen-ounce Pepsi."

I looked at the list. "To tell you the truth, Fats, I'm afraid to add it all up," I said. I looked at the list again. Something on it had reminded me of Italian sausages. I decided that I would walk over to the fair later and have just one sausage sandwich with peppers and onions— saving a few calories by having a barbecued rather than a fried sausage. If things got out of hand, I figured, I could always go on one of those diets that allow you as much as you want to eat as long as you eat only Brussels sprouts, quinces, and summer squash. I had mentioned the fair to Fats, but he couldn't go. It wasn't a Monday.

"Is life worth living, Fats?" I asked.

"Well, I figure that in my first twenty-five years I ate enough for four normal lifetimes," Fats said. "So I get along. But there is a lot of pain involved. A lot of pain. I can't stress that enough."

STARTING ON MONDAY

by Judith Viorst

Starting on Monday I'm living on carrots and bouillon.
Starting on Monday I'm bidding the bagel adieu.
I'm switching from Hersheys with almonds to gaunt and
    anemic,
And people will ask me could that skinny person be you.
I'll count every calorie from squash (half a cup, 47)
To Life Saver (8), stalk of celery (5), pepper ring (2),
Starting on Monday.

Starting on Monday I'll jog for a mile in the morning.
(That's after the sit-ups and push-ups and touching my toes.)
The gratification I once used to seek in lasagna
I'll find on the day that I have to go buy smaller clothes.
I'll turn my attention from infantile pleasures like Clark Bars
To things like the song of a bird and the scent of a rose.
Starting on Monday.

Starting on Monday my will will be stronger than brownies,
And anything more than an unsalted egg will seem crude.
My inner-thigh fat and my upper-arm flab will diminish.
My cheeks will be hollowed, my ribs will begin to protrude.
The bones of my pelvis will make their initial appearance—
A testament to my relentless abstention from food,
Starting on Monday.

But Tuesday a friend came for coffee and brought homemade
    muffins.
And Wednesday I had to quit jogging because of my back.

On Thursday I read in the paper an excess of egg yolk
Would clog up my vessels and certainly cause an attack.
On Friday we ate at the Goldfarbs'. She always makes cream
    sauce,
And always gets sulky if people don't eat what she makes.
On Saturday evening we went with the kids to a drive-in.
I begged for a Fresca but all they were selling were shakes.
On Sunday my stomach oozed over the top of my waistband,
And filled with self-loathing I sought consolation in pie
And the thought that Onassis could bribe me with yachts and
    with emeralds
But still I'd refuse to taste even a single French fry . . .
Starting on Monday.

THE ECHO AND THE NEMESIS

by Jean Stafford

Sue Ledbetter and Ramona Dunn became friends through the commonplace accident of their sitting side by side in a philosophy lecture three afternoons a week. There were many other American students at Heidelberg University that winter—the last before the war—but neither Sue nor Ramona had taken up with them. Ramona had not because she scorned them; in her opinion, they were Philistines, concerned only with drinking beer, singing German songs, and making spectacles of themselves on their bicycles and in their little rented cars. And Sue had not because she was self-conscious and introverted and did not make friends easily. In Ramona's presence, she pretended to deplore her compatriots' escapades, which actually she envied desperately. Sometimes on Saturday nights she lay on her bed unable to read or daydream and in an agony of frustration as she listened to her fellow-lodgers at the Pension Kirchenheim laughing and teasing and sometimes bursting into song as they played bridge and Monopoly in the cozy veranda café downstairs.

Soon after the semester opened in October, the two girls fell into the habit of drinking their afternoon coffee together on the days they met in class. Neither of them especially enjoyed the other's company, but in their different ways they were lonely, and as Ramona once remarked, in her highfalutin way, "From time to time, I need a rest from the exercitation of my intellect." She was very vain of her intellect, which she had directed to the study of philology, to the exclusion of almost everything else in the world. Sue, while she had always taken her work seriously, longed also for beaux and parties, and conversation about them, and she was often bored by Ramona's talk, obscurely gossipy, of the vagaries of certain Old High Franconian verbs when they encountered the High German consonant shift, or of the variant readings of passages in Layamon's *Brut,* or the linguistic influence Eleanor of Aquitaine had exerted on the English court. But because she was well-mannered she listened politely and even appeared to follow Ramona's exuberant elucidation of Sanskrit "a"-stem declensions and her ardent plan to write a monograph on the word "ahoy." They drank their coffee in the Konditorei Luitpold, a very noisy café on a street bent like an elbow, down behind the cathedral. The din of its two small rooms was aggravated by the peripheral racket that came from the kitchen and from the outer shop, where the cakes were kept. The waiters, all of whom looked cross, hustled about at a great rate, slamming down trays and glasses and cups any which way before the many customers, who gabbled and rattled newspapers and pounded on the table for more of something. Over all the to-do was the blare of the radio, with its dial set permanently at a station that played nothing but stormy choruses from *Wilhelm Tell.* Ramona, an invincible expositor, had to shout, but shout she did as she traced words like "rope" and "calf" through dozens of languages back to their Indo-Germanic source. Sometimes Sue, befuddled by the uproar, wanted by turns to laugh and to cry with disappointment, for this was not at all the way she had imagined that she would live in Europe. Half incredulously and half irritably, she would stare at Ramona as if in some way she were to blame.

Ramona Dunn was fat to the point of parody. Her obesity fitted her badly, like extra clothing put on in the wintertime, for her embedded bones were very small and she was very short, and she had a foolish gait, which, however, was swift, as if she were a mechanical doll whose engine raced. Her face was rather pretty, but its features were so small that it was all but lost in its billowing surroundings, and it was covered by a thin, fair skin that was subject to disfiguring affections, now hives, now eczema, now impetigo, and the whole was framed by fine, pale hair that was abused once a week by a *Friseur* who baked it with an iron into dozens of horrid little snails. She habitually wore a crimson tam-o'-shanter with a sportive spray of artificial edelweiss pinned to the very top of it. For so determined a bluestocking, her eccentric and extensive wardrobe was a surprise; nothing was ever completely clean or completely whole, and nothing ever matched anything else, but it was apparent that all these odd and often ugly clothes had been expensive. She had a long, fur-lined cape, and men's tweed jackets with leather patches on the elbows, and flannel shirts designed for hunters in the state of Maine, and high-necked jerseys, and a waistcoat made of unborn gazelle, dyed Kelly green. She attended particularly to the dressing of her tiny hands and feet, and she had gloves and mittens of every color and every material, and innumerable pairs of extraordinary shoes, made for her by a Roman boot-maker. She always carried a pair of field glasses, in a brass-bound leather case that hung over her shoulder by a plaited strap of rawhide; she looked through the wrong end of them, liking, for some reason that she did not disclose, to diminish the world she surveyed. Wherever she went, she took a locked pigskin satchel, in which she carried her grammars and lexicons and the many drafts of the many articles she was writing in the hope that they would be published in learned journals. One day in the café, soon after the girls became acquainted, she opened up the satchel, and Sue was shocked at the helter-skelter arrangement of the papers, all mussed and frayed, and stained with coffee and ink. But, even more, she was dumfounded to see a clear-green all-day sucker stuck like a bookmark between the pages of a glossary to *Beowulf.*

Sue knew that Ramona was rich, and that for the last ten years her family had lived in Italy, and that before that they had lived in New York. But this was all she knew about her friend; she did not even know where she lived in Heidelberg. She believed that Ramona, in her boundless erudition, was truly consecrated to her studies and that she truly had no other desire than to impress the subscribers to *Speculum* and the *Publications of the Modern Language Association*. She was the sort of person who seemed, at twenty-one, to have fought all her battles and survived to enjoy the quiet of her unendangered ivory tower. She did not seem to mind at all that she was so absurd to look at, and Sue, who was afire with ambitions and sick with conflict, admired her arrogant self-possession.

The two girls had been going to the Konditorei Luitpold three times a week for a month or more, and all these meetings had been alike; Ramona had talked and Sue had contributed expressions of surprise (who would have dreamed that "bolster" and "poltroon" derived from the same parent?), or murmurs of acquiescence (she agreed there might be something in the discreet rumor that the Gothic language had been made up by nineteenth-century scholars to answer riddles that could not otherwise be solved), or laughter, when it seemed becoming. The meetings were neither rewarding nor entirely uninteresting to Sue, and she came to look upon them as a part of the week's schedule, like the philosophy lectures and the seminar in Schiller.

And then, one afternoon, just as the weary, mean-mouthed waiter set their cake down before them, the radio departed from its custom and over it came the "Minuet in G," so neat and winning and surprising that for a moment there was a general lull in the café, and even the misanthropic waiter paid the girls the honor, in his short-lived delight, of not slopping their coffee. As if they all shared the same memories that the little sentimental piece of music awoke in her, Sue glanced around smiling at her fellows and tried to believe that all of them—even the old men with Hindenburg mustaches and palsied wattles, and even the Brown Shirts fiercely playing chess—had been children like herself and had stumbled in buckled pumps through the simple steps of the minuet at the military command of a dancing teacher, Miss Conklin, who had bared her sinewy

legs to the thigh. In some public presentation of Miss Conklin's class, Sue had worn a yellow bodice with a lacing of
black velvet ribbon, a bouffant skirt of chintz covered all
over with daffodils, and a cotton-batting wig that smelled
of stale talcum powder. Even though her partner had been
a sissy boy with nastily damp hands and white eyelashes,
and though she had been grave with stage fright, she had
had moments of most thrilling expectation, as if this were
only the dress rehearsal of the grown-up ball to come.

If she had expected all the strangers in the café to be
transported by the "Minuet" to a sweet and distant time,
she had not expected Ramona Dunn to be, and she was
astonished and oddly frightened to see the fat girl gazing
with a sad, reflective smile into her water glass. When the
music stopped and the familiar hullabaloo was reestab-
lished in the room, Ramona said, "Oh, I don't know of
anything that makes me more nostalgic than that tinny little
tune! It makes me think of Valentine parties before my
sister Martha died."

It took Sue a minute to rearrange her family portrait of
the Dunns, which heretofore had included, besides Ramona, only a mother and a father and three brothers. Because this was by far the simplest way, she had seen them
in her mind's eye as five stout, scholarly extensions of Ramona, grouped together against the background of Vesuvius. She had imagined that they spent their time examining
papyri and writing Latin verses, and she regretted admit-
ting sorrow into their lives, as she had to do when she saw
Ramona's eyes grow vague and saw her, quite unlike her
naturally greedy self, push her cake aside, untouched. For
a moment or two, the fat girl was still and blank, as if she
were waiting for a pain to go away, and then she poured
the milk into her coffee, replaced her cake, and began to
talk about her family, who, it seemed, were not in the least
as Sue had pictured them.

Ramona said that she alone of them was fat and ill-
favored, and the worst of it was that Martha, the most
beautiful girl who ever lived, had been her twin. Sue could

not imagine, she declared, how frightfully good-looking all the Dunns were—except herself, of course: tall and dark-eyed and oval-faced, and tanned from the hours they spent on their father's boat, the *San Filippo*. And they were terribly gay and venturesome; they were the despair of the croupiers at the tables on the Riviera, the envy of the skiers at San Bernardino and of the yachtsmen on the Mediterranean. Their balls and their musicales and their dinner parties were famous. All the brothers had unusual artistic gifts, and there was so much money in the family that they did not have to do anything but work for their own pleasure in their studios. They were forever involved in scandals with their mistresses, who were either married noble-women or notorious dancing girls, and forever turning over a new leaf and getting themselves engaged to lovely, convent-bred princesses, whom, however, they did not marry; the young ladies were too submissively Catholic, or too stupid, or their taste in painting was vulgar.

Of all this charming, carefree brood, Martha, five years dead, had been the most splendid, Ramona said, a creature so slight and delicate that one wanted to put her under a glass bell to protect her. Painters were captivated by the elegant shape of her head, around which she wore her chestnut hair in a coronet, and there were a dozen portraits of her, and hundreds of drawings hanging in the big bedroom where she had died and which now had been made into a sort of shrine for her. If the Dunns were odd in any way, it was in this devotion to their dead darling; twice a year Mrs. Dunn changed the nibs in Martha's pens, and in one garden there grew nothing but anemones, Martha's favorite flower. She had ailed from birth, pursued malevolently by the disease that had melted her away to the wick finally when she was sixteen. The family had come to Italy in the beginning of her mortal languor in the hope that the warmth and novelty would revive her, and for a while it did, but the wasting poison continued to devour her slowly, and for years she lay, a touching invalid, on a balcony overlooking the Bay of Naples. She lay on a blond satin chaise longue, in a quaint peignoir made of leaf-green velvet, and sometimes, as she regarded her prospect of sloops and valiant skiffs on the turbulent waves, the cypress trees, white villas in the midst of olive groves, the intransigent smoldering of Vesuvius, she sang old English airs and Irish songs as she accompanied herself on a lute. If, in the erratic course of her illness, she got a little stronger, she asked for extra cushions at her back and half sat up at a small easel to paint in water-colors, liking the volcano as a subject, trite as it was, and the comic tourist boats that romped over the bay from Naples to Capri. If she was very unwell, she simply lay smiling while her parents and her sister and her brothers attended her, trying to seduce her back to health with their futile offerings of plums and tangerines and gilt-stemmed glasses of Rhine wine and nosegays bought from the urchins who bargained on the carriage roads.

When Martha died, Ramona's own grief was despair, because the death of a twin is a foretaste of one's own death, and for months she had been harried with premonitions and prophetic dreams, and often she awoke to find that she had strayed from her bed, for what awful purpose she did not know, and was walking barefoot, like a pilgrim, down the pitch-black road. But the acute phase of her mourning had passed, and now, although sorrow was always with her, like an alter ego, she had got over the worst of it.

She paused in her narrative and unexpectedly laughed. "What a gloom I'm being!" she said, and resumed her monologue at once but in a lighter tone, this time to recount the drubbing her brother Justin had given someone when he was defending the honor of a dishonorable soprano, and to suggest, in tantalizing innuendoes, that her parents were not faithful to each other.

Sue, whose dead father had been an upright, pessimistic clergyman and whose mother had never given voice to an impure thought, was bewitched by every word Ramona said. It occurred to her once to wonder why Ramona so frowned upon the frolics of the other American students when her beloved relatives were so worldly, but then she realized that the manners of the *haut monde* were one thing and those of undergraduates another. How queer, Sue thought, must seem this freakish bookworm in the midst of it all! And yet such was the ease with which Ramona talked, so exquisitely placed were her fillips of French, so intimate and casual her allusions to the rich and celebrated figures of international society, that Ramona changed before Sue's eyes; from the envelope of fat emerged a personality as *spirituelle* and knowing as any practicing sophisticate's. When, in the course of describing a distiller from Milan who was probably her mother's lover, she broke off and pressingly issued Sue an invitation to go with her a month from then, at the Christmas holiday, to San Bernardino to meet her brothers for a fortnight of skiing, Sue accepted immediately, not stopping to think, in the heady pleasure of the moment, that the proposal was unduly sudden, considering the sketchy nature of their friendship. "My brothers will adore you," she said, giving Sue a look of calm appraisal. "They are eclectic and they'll find your red hair and brown eyes irresistibly naïve." As if the plan had long been in her mind, Ramona named the date they would leave Heidelberg; she begged permission, in the most gracious and subtlest possible way, to let Sue be her guest, even to the extent of supplying her with ski equipment. When the details were settled—a little urgently, she made Sue promise "on her word of honor" that she would not default—she again took up her report on Signor de Gama, the distiller, who was related by blood to the Pope and had other distinctions of breeding as well to recommend him to her mother, who was, she confessed, something of a snob. "Mama," she said, accenting the ultima, "thinks it is unnecessary for anyone to be badly born."

The Konditorei Luitpold was frequented by teachers from the Translators' Institute, and usually Ramona rejoiced in listening to them chattering and expostulating, in half a dozen European languages, for she prided herself on her gift of tongues. But today her heart was in Sorrento, and she paid no attention to them, not even to two vociferous young Russians at a table nearby. She disposed of the roué from Milan (Sue had read Catullus? Signor da Gama had a cottage at Sirmio not far from his reputed grave) and seemed to be on the point of disclosing her father's delinquencies when she was checked by a new mood, which made her lower her head, flush, and, through a long moment of silence, study the greasy hoops the rancid milk had made on the surface of her coffee.

Sue felt as if she had inadvertently stumbled upon a scene of deepest privacy, which, if she were not careful, she would violate, and, pretending that she had not observed the hiatus at all, she asked, conversationally, the names of Ramona's brothers besides Justin.

The two others were called Daniel and Robert, but it was not of them, or of her parents, or of Martha, that Ramona now wanted to speak but of herself, and haltingly she said that the "Minuet in G" had deranged her poise because it had made her think of the days of her childhood in New York, when she had been no bigger than her twin and they had danced the minuet together, Ramona taking the dandy's part. A friend of the family had predicted that though they were then almost identical, Ramona was going to be the prettier of the two. Now Sue was shocked, for she had thought that Ramona must always have been fat, and she was nearly moved to tears to know that the poor girl had been changed from a swan into an ugly duckling and that it was improbable, from the looks of her, that she would ever be changed back again. But Sue was so young and so badly equipped to console someone so beset that she could not utter a word, and she wished she could go home.

Ramona summoned the waiter and ordered her third piece of cake, saying nervously, after she had done so, "I'm sorry. When I get upset, I have to eat to calm myself. I'm awful! I ought to kill myself for eating so much." She began to devour the cake obsessively, and when she had finished it down to the last crumb, and the last fragment of frosting, she said, with shimmering eyes, "Please let me tell you what it is that makes me the unhappiest girl in the world, and maybe you can help me." Did Sue have any idea what it was like to be ruled by food and half driven out of one's mind until one dreamed of it and had at last no other ambition but to eat incessantly with an appetite that grew and grew until one saw oneself, in nightmares, as nothing but an enormous mouth and a tongue, trembling lasciviously? Did she know the terror and the remorse that followed on the heels of it when one slyly sneaked the lion's share of buttered toast at tea? Had she ever desired the whole of a pudding meant for twelve and hated with all her heart the others at the dinner table? Sue could not hide her blushing face or put her fingers in her ears or close her eyes against the tortured countenance of that wretched butterball, who declared that she had often come within an ace of doing away with herself because she was so fat.

Leaning across the table, almost whispering, Ramona went on, "I didn't come to Heidelberg for its philologists—they don't know any more than I do. I have exiled myself. I would not any longer offend that long-suffering family of mine with the sight of me." It had been her aim to fast throughout this year, she continued, and return to them transformed, and she had hoped to be thinner by many pounds when she joined her brothers at Christmastime. But she had at once run into difficulties, because, since she was not altogether well (she did not specify her illness and Sue would not have asked its name for anything), she had to be under the supervision of a doctor. And the doctor in Heidelberg, like the doctor in Naples, would not take her seriously when she said her fatness was ruining her life; they had both gone so far as to say that she was *meant* to be like this and that it would be imprudent of her to diet. Who was bold enough to fly in the face of medical authority? Not she, certainly.

It appeared, did it not, to be a dilemma past solution, Ramona asked. And yet this afternoon she had begun to see a way out, if Sue would pledge herself to help. Sue did not reply at once, sensing an involvement, but then she thought of Ramona's brothers, whom she was going to please, and she said she would do what she could.

"You're not just saying that? You are my friend? You know, of course, that you'll be repaid a hundredfold." Ramona subjected Sue's sincerity to some minutes of investigation and then outlined her plan, which seemed very tame to Sue after all these preparations, for it consisted only of Ramona's defying Dr. Freudenburg and of Sue's becoming a sort of unofficial censor and confessor. Sue was to have lunch with her each day, at Ramona's expense, and was to remind her, by a nudge or a word now and again, not to eat more than was really necessary to keep alive. If at any time Sue suspected that she was eating between meals or late at night, she was to come out flatly with an accusation and so shame Ramona that it would never happen again. The weekends were particularly difficult, since there were no lectures to go to and it was tempting not to stir out of her room at all but to gorge throughout the day on delicacies out of tins and boxes that she had sent to herself from shops in Strasbourg and Berlin. And since, in addition to fasting, she needed exercise, she hoped that Sue would agree to go walking with her on Saturdays and Sundays, a routine that could be varied from time to time by a weekend trip to some neighboring town of interest.

When Sue protested mildly that Ramona had contradicted her earlier assertion that she would not dare dispute her doctor's word, Ramona grinned roguishly and said only, "Don't be nosy."

Ramona had found an old ladies' home, called the Gerstnerheim, which, being always in need of funds, welcomed paying guests at the midday meal, whom they fed for a unimaginably low price. Ramona did not patronize it out of miserliness, however, but because the food was nearly inedible. And it was here that the girls daily took their Spartan lunch. It was quite the worst food that Sue had ever eaten anywhere, for it was cooked to pallor and flaccidity and then was seasoned with unheard-of condiments, which sometimes made her sick. The bread was sour and the soup was full of pasty clots; the potatoes were waterlogged and the old red cabbage was boiled until it was blue. The dessert was always a basin of molded farina with a sauce of gray jelly that had a gray taste. The aged ladies sat at one enormously long table, preserving an institutional silence until the farina was handed around, and as if this were an alarm, all the withered lips began to move simultaneously and from them issued high squawks of protest against the dreary lot of being old and homeless and underfed. Sue could not help admiring Ramona, who ate her plate of eel and celeriac as if she really preferred it to tuna broiled with black olives and who talked all the while of things quite other than food—of Walther von der Vogelweide's eccentric syntax, of a new French novel that had come in the mail that morning, and of their trip to Switzerland.

Justin and Daniel and Robert were delighted that Sue was coming, Ramona said, and arrangements were being made in a voluminous correspondence through the air over the Alps. Sue had never been on skis in her life, but she did not allow this to deflate her high hopes. She thought only of evenings of lieder (needless to say, the accomplished Dunns sang splendidly) and hot spiced wine before a dancing fire, of late breakfasts in the white sun and brilliant conversation. And of what was coming afterward! The later holidays (Ramona called them *villeggiatura*), spent in Sorrento! The countesses' garden parties in Amalfi and the cruises on the Adriatic, the visits to Greece, the balls in the princely houses of Naples! Ramona could not decide which of her brothers Sue would elect to marry. Probably Robert, she thought, since he was the youngest and the most affectionate.

It was true that Sue did not quite believe all she was told, but she knew that the ways of the rich are strange, and while she did not allow her fantasies to invade the hours assigned to classes and study, she did not rebuff them when they came at moments of leisure. From time to time, she suddenly remembered that she was required to give something in return for Ramona's largess, and then she would say how proud she was of her friend's self-discipline or would ask her, like a frank and compassionate doctor, if she had strayed at all from her intention (she always had; she always immediately admitted it and Sue always put on a show of disappointment), and once in a while she said that Ramona was looking much thinner, although this was absolutely untrue. Sometimes they took the electric tram to Neckargemünd, where they split a bottle of sweet Greek wine. Occasionally they went to Mannheim, to the opera, but they never stayed for a full performance; Ramona said that later in the year Signor de Gama would invite them to his house in Milan and then they could go to La Scala every night. Once they went for a weekend to Rothenburg, where Ramona, in an uncontrollable holiday mood, ate twelve cherry tarts in a single day. She was tearful for a week afterward, and to show Sue how sorry she was, she ground out a cigarette on one of her downy wrists. This dreadful incident took place in the Luitpold and was witnessed by several patrons, who could not conceal their alarm. Sue thought to herself, Maybe she's cuckoo, and while she did not relinquish any of her daydreams of the festivities in Italy, she began to observe Ramona more closely.

Sue could feel the turmoil in her when they went past bakeshop windows full of cream puffs and cheesecake and petits fours. Ramona, furtively glancing at the goodies out of the corner of her eye, would begin a passionate and long-winded speech on the present-day use of Latin in Iceland. When, on a special occasion, they dined together at the Ritterhalle, she did not even look at the menu but lionheartedly ordered a single dropped egg and a cup of tea and resolutely kept her eyes away from Sue's boiled beef and fritters. When drinking cocktails in the American bar at the Europäischer Hof, she shook her head as the waiter passed a tray of canapés made of caviar, anchovy, lobster, foie gras, and Camembert, ranged fanwise around a little bowl of ivory almonds. But sometimes she did capitulate, with a piteous rationalization—that she had not eaten any breakfast or that she had barely touched her soup at the Gerstnerheim and that therefore there would be nothing wrong in her having two or perhaps three or four of these tiny little sandwiches. One time Sue saw her take several more than she had said she would and hide them under the rim of her plate.

As the date set for their departure for Switzerland drew nearer, Ramona grew unaccountable. Several times she failed to appear at lunch, and when Sue, in a friendly way, asked for an explanation, she snapped, "None of your business. What do you think you are? My nurse?" She was full of peevishness, complaining of the smell of senility in the Gerstnerheim, of students who sucked the shells of pistachio nuts in the library, of her landlady's young son, who she was sure rummaged through her bureau drawers when she was not at home. Once she and Sue had a fearful row when Sue, keeping up her end of the bargain, although she really did not care a pin, told her not to buy a bag of chestnuts from a vendor on a street corner. Ramona shouted, for all the world to hear, "You are sadly mistaken, Miss Ledbetter, if you think you know more than Dr. Augustus Freudenburg, of the Otto-Ludwigs Clinic!" And a little after that she acquired the notion that people were staring at her, and she carried an umbrella, rain or shine, to hide herself from them. But, oddest of all, when the skis and boots and poles that she had ordered for Sue arrived, and Sue thanked her for them, she said, "I can't think what use they'll be. Obviously there never is any snow in this ghastly, godforsaken place."

There was an awful afternoon when Ramona was convinced that the waiter at the Luitpold had impugned her German, and Sue found herself in the unhappy role of intermediary in a preposterous altercation so bitter that it stopped just short of a bodily engagement. When the girls left the café—at the insistence of the management—they were silent all the way to the cathedral, which was the place where they usually took leave of each other to go their separate ways home. They paused a moment there in the growing dark, and suddenly Ramona said, "Look at me!" Sue looked at her. "I say!" said Ramona. "In this light you look exactly like my sister. How astonishing! Turn a little to the left, there's a dear." And when Sue had turned as she directed, a whole minute—but it seemed an hour to Sue—passed before Ramona broke from her trance to cry, "How blind I've been! My brothers would be shocked to death if they should see you. It would kill them!"

She put out her hands, on which she wore white leather mittens, and held Sue's face between them and studied it, half closing her eyes and murmuring her amazement, her delight, her perplexity at her failure until now to see this marvelous resemblance. Once, as her brown eyes nimbly catechized the face before her, she took off her right mitten and ran her index finger down Sue's nose, as if she had even learned her sister's bones by heart, while Sue, unable to speak, could only think in panic, What does she mean *if* they should see me?

Ramona carried on as if she were moon-struck, making fresh discoveries until not only were Sue's and Martha's faces identical but so were their voices and their carriage and the shape of their hands and feet. She said, "You must come to my room and see a picture of Martha right now. It's desperately weird."

Fascinated, Sue nodded, and they moved on through the quiet street. Ramona paused to look at her each time they went under a street light, touched her hair, begged leave to take her arm, and called her Martha, Sister, Twin, and sometimes caught her breath in an abortive sob. They went past the lighted windows of the *Bierstuben,* where the shadows of young men loomed and waved, and then turned at the Kornmarkt and began to climb the steep, moss-slick steps that led to the castle garden. As they went through the avenue of trees that lay between the casino and the castle, Ramona, peering at Sue through the spooky mist, said, "They would have been much quicker to see it than I," so Sue knew, miserably and for sure, that something had gone wrong with their plans to go to San Bernardino. And then Ramona laughed and broke away and took off her tam-o'-shanter, which she hurled toward the hedge of yew, where it rested tipsily.

"I could vomit," she said, standing absolutely still.

There was a long pause. Finally, Sue could no longer bear the suspense, and she asked Ramona if her brothers knew that she and Ramona were not coming.

"Of course they know. They've known for two weeks, but you're crazy if you think the reason we're not going is that you look like Martha. How beastly vain you are!" She was so angry and she trembled so with her rage that Sue did not dare say another word. "It was Freudenburg who said I couldn't go," she howled. "He has found out that I have lost ten pounds."

Sue had no conscious motive in asking her, idly and not really caring, where Dr. Freudenburg's office was; she had meant the guileless question to be no more than a show of noncommittal and courteous interest, and she was badly frightened when, in reply, Ramona turned on her and slapped her hard on either cheek, and then opened her mouth to emit one hideous, protracted scream. Sue started instinctively to run away, but Ramona seized and held her arms, and began to talk in a lunatic, fast monotone, threatening her with lawsuits and public exposure if she ever mentioned the name Freudenburg again *or* her brothers *or* her mother and father *or* Martha, that ghastly, puling, pampered hypochondriac who had totally wrecked her life.

Sue felt that the racket of her heart and her hot, prancing brain would drown out Ramona's voice, but it did nothing of the kind, and they stood there, rocking in their absurd attitude, while the fit continued. Sue was sure that the police and the townsfolk would come running at any moment and an alarm would be sounded and they would be arrested for disturbing the peace. But if anyone heard them, it was only the shades of the princes in the castle.

It was difficult for Sue to sort out the heroes and the villains in this diatribe. Sometimes it appeared that Ramona's brothers and her parents hated her, sometimes she thought they had been glad when Martha died; sometimes Dr. Freudenburg seemed to be the cause of everything. She had the impression that he was an alienist, and she wondered if now he would send his patient to an institution; at other times she thought the doctor did not exist at all. She did not know whom to hate or whom to trust, for the characters in this *Walpurgisnacht* changed shape by the minute and not a one was left out—not Signor da Gama or the ballet girls in Naples or the old ladies at the Gerstnerheim or the prehistoric figures of a sadistic nurse, a base German governess, and a nefarious boy cousin who had invited Ramona to misbehave when she was barely eight years old. Once she said that to escape Dr. Freudenburg she meant to order her father to take her cruising on the *San Filippo;* a minute later she said that that loathsome fool Justin had wrecked the boat on the coast of Yugoslavia. She would go home to the villa in Sorrento and be comforted by her brothers who had always preferred her to everyone else in the world—except that they hadn't! They had always despised her. Freudenburg would write to her father and he would come to fetch her back to that vulgar, parvenu house, and there, in spite of all her efforts to outwit them, they would make her eat and eat until she was the laughing stock of the entire world. What *were* they after? Did they want to indenture her to a sideshow?

She stopped, trailed off, turned loose Sue's arm, and stood crestfallen, like a child who realizes that no one is listening to his tantrum. Tears, terribly silent, streamed down her round cheeks.

Then, "It isn't true, you know. They aren't like that, they're good and kind. The only thing that's true is that I eat all the time," and softly, to herself, she repeated, "All the time." In a mixture of self-hatred and abstracted bravado, she said that she had supplemented all her lunches at the Gerstnerheim and had nibbled constantly, alone in her room; that Dr. Freudenburg's recommendation had been just the opposite of what she had been saying all along.

Unconsolable, Ramona moved on along the path, and Sue followed, honoring her tragedy but struck dumb by it. On the way through the courtyard and down the street, Ramona told her, in a restrained and rational voice, that her father was coming the next day to take her back to Italy, since the experiment of her being here alone had not worked. Her parents, at the counsel of Dr. Freudenburg, were prepared to take drastic measures, involving, if need be, a hospital, the very thought of which made her blood run cold. "Forgive me for that scene back there," she said. "You grow wild in loneliness like mine. It would have been lovely if it had all worked out the way I wanted and we had gone to Switzerland."

"Oh, that's all right," said Sue, whose heart was broken. "I don't know how to ski anyway."

"Really? What crust! I'd never have bought you all that gear if I had known." Ramona laughed lightly. They approached the garden gate of a tall yellow house, and she said, "This is where I live. Want to come in and have a glass of kirsch?"

Sue did not want the kirsch and she knew she should be on her way home if she were to get anything hot for supper, but she was curious to see the photograph of Martha, and since Ramona seemed herself again, she followed her down the path. Ramona had two little rooms, as clean and orderly as cells. In the one where she studied, there was no furniture except a long desk with deep drawers and a straight varnished chair and a listing bookcase. She had very few books, really, for one so learned—not more than fifty altogether—and every one of them was dull: grammars, dictionaries, readers, monographs reprinted from scholarly journals, and treatises on semantics, etymology, and phonetics. Her pens and pencils lay straight in a lacquered tray, and a pile of notebooks sat neatly at the right of the blotter, and at the left there was a book open to a homily in Anglo-Saxon which, evidently, she had been translating. As soon as they had taken off their coats, Ramona went into the bedroom and closed the door; from beyond it Sue could hear drawers being opened and quickly closed, metal clashing, and paper rustling, and she imagined that the bureaus were stocked with contraband—with sweets and sausages and cheese. For the last time, she thought of Daniel and Justin and Robert, of whom she was to be forever deprived because their sister could not curb her brutish appetite.

She wandered around the room and presently her eye fell on a photograph in a silver frame standing in a half-empty shelf of the bookcase. It could only be Martha. The dead girl did not look in the least like Sue but was certainly as pretty as she had been described, and as Sue looked at the pensive eyes and the thoughtful lips, she was visited by a fugitive feeling that this was really Ramona's face at which she looked and that it had been refined and made immaculate by an artful photographer who did not scruple to help his clients deceive themselves. For Martha wore a look of lovely wonder and remoteness, as if she were all disconnected spirit, and it was the same as a look that sometimes came to Ramona's eyes and lips just as she lifted her binoculars to contemplate the world through the belittling lenses.

Sue turned the photograph around, and on the back she read the penned inscription "Martha Ramona Dunn at sixteen, Sorrento." She looked at that ethereal face again, and this time had no doubt that it had once belonged to Ramona. No wonder the loss of it had left her heartbroken! She sighed to think of her friend's desperate fabrication. In a sense, she supposed the Martha side of Ramona Dunn *was* dead, dead and buried under layers and layers of fat. Just as she guiltily returned the picture to its place, the door to the bedroom opened and Ramona, grandly gesturing toward her dressing table, cried, "Come in! Come in! Enter the banquet hall!" She had emptied the drawers of all their forbidden fruits, and arrayed on the dressing table, in front of her bottles of cologne and medicine, were cheeses and tinned fish and pickles and pressed meat and cakes, candies, nuts, olives, sausages, buns, apples, raisins, figs, prunes, dates, and jars of pâté and glasses of jelly and little pots of caviar, as black as ink. "Don't stint!" she shouted, and she bounded forward and began to eat as if she had not had a meal in weeks.

"All evidence must be removed by morning! What a close shave! What if my father had come without telling me and had found it all!" Shamelessly, she ranged up and down the table, cropping and lowing like a cow in a pasture. There were droplets of sweat on her forehead and her hands were shaking, but nothing else about her showed that she had gone to pieces earlier or that she was deep, deeper by far than anyone else Sue had ever known.

Sucking a rind of citron, Ramona said, "You must realize that our friendship is over, but not through any fault of yours. When I went off and turned on you that way, it had nothing to do with you at all, for of course you don't look any more like Martha than the man in the moon."

"It's all right, Ramona," said Sue politely. She stayed close to the door, although the food looked very good. "I'll still be your friend."

"Oh, no, no, there would be nothing in it for you," Ramona said, and her eyes narrowed ever so slightly. "Thank you just the same. I am exceptionally ill." She spoke with pride, as if she were really saying "I am exceptionally talented" or "I am exceptionally attractive."

"I didn't know you were," said Sue. "I'm sorry."

"*I'm* not sorry. It is for yourself that you should be sorry. You have such a trivial little life, poor girl. It's not your fault. Most people do."

"I'd better go," said Sue.

"Go! Go!" cried Ramona, with a gesture of grand benediction. "I weep not."

Sue's hand was on the knob of the outer door, but she hesitated to leave a scene so inconclusive. Ramona watched her as she lingered; her mouth was so full that her cheeks were stretched out as if in mumps, and through the food and through a devilish, mad grin she said, "Of *course* you could never know the divine joy of being twins, provincial one! Do you know what he said the last night when my name was Martha? The night he came into that room where the anemones were? He pretended that he was looking for a sheet of music. Specifically for a sonata for the harpsichord by Wilhelm Friedrich Bach."

But Sue did not wait to hear what he, whoever he was, had said; she ran down the brown-smelling stairs and out into the cold street with the feeling that Ramona was still standing there before the food, as if she were serving herself at an altar, still talking, though there was no one to listen. She wondered if she ought to summon Dr. Freudenburg, and then decided that, in the end, it was none of her business. She caught a trolley that took her near her pension, and was just in time to get some hot soup and a plate of cold meats and salad before the kitchen closed. But when the food came, she found that she had no appetite at all. "What's the matter?" asked Herr Sachs, the fresh young waiter. "Are you afraid to get fat?" And he looked absolutely flabbergasted when, at this, she fled from the café without a word.

Note

When I wrote this story, I did not know that dogged secret nibbling and secret sprees of gorging were symptoms of an accredited neurosis which had been studied and described for years in psychiatric journals. I was, indeed, so backward that I thought obesity—save when the cause of it was glandular—was punishment for the deadly sin of Gluttony. Today, when throughout the length and breadth of the land there are almost as many cells for Weight Watchers as there are for Alcoholics Anonymous, I might have struck a different chord. I am glad I did not know what the doctors and their tortured patients knew, for if I had, I would have been inhibited, fearing, on the one hand, that I might not parse medically and, on the other, that I might smell of the clinic. Once, long before I ever conceived the character of Ramona Dunn, when I was morbidly leafing through a textbook for first-year medical students, I came upon the photograph of a woman afflicted, so the caption read, with *adiposis dolorosa* and I think that "sorrowful fat" must have stuck in my mind and that the adjective led to my invention of Ramona's despair and her concealing, consoling paranoia.

It has been thought that I wrote autobigraphically and not long after the story was published, I was considerably taken aback to receive in the mail reprints of two lectures, one on some of the reasons for overeating, the other on the ordeals and the pitfalls and the occasional rewards of dieting, both signed by the psychiatrist who had delivered them and who, in an accompanying note, expressed a willingness to see me some time in June when his schedule would be more flexible than usual. Finding this drumming up of trade importunate and shamefully unprofessional, I inquired into the man's credentials and, on learning that they were immaculate, concluded that he had read between my lines—but had done so astigmatically because of his preoccupation—and judged that my struggle against adiposity was so dolorous that he wanted to lend a hand out of the goodness of his heart. Having no need to do so, I did not reply. If I *had* been writing confessionally, I would have been hindered in another way: if I *had* been Ramona, resentment would have befogged my vision and self-contempt would have tricked me into burlesque.

To the writer of fiction, a little learning of Freud's hypotheses and those of his successors isn't seriously dangerous. More, however, is; and much is disastrous.

—*Jean Stafford*

THE FOOD FARM

By **Kit Reed**

*I had already written one fat story, "The Fat Sisters," when
I met Jean Stafford, but that didn't seem to be the end of
it. I was enthralled by newspaper accounts of life at Maine
Chance, the posh resort where rich ladies paid thousands
to have pounds starved and pounded off. Miss Stafford,
who had published "The Echo and the Nemesis" some
years before we met, shared some of my fascination, offering some wonderful bits of gossip. In time I went on to
write "The Food Farm," and it was not until I reread "The
Echo and the Nemesis" some years later that I realized how
big my debt to Jean Stafford was. I had even gone so far
as to name my second fat girl "Ramona," and I had given
her a family background similar to that of Ramona Dunn—
right down to the family yacht. So herewith, with all credit
due: "The Food Farm."*

*Introducing this story in one of her anthologies, Judith
Merril said it in print: "Inside every thin woman, there is
a fat one, screaming. . ."*

So here I am, warden-in-charge, fattening them up for our
leader, Tommy Fango; here I am laying on the banana
pudding and the milkshakes and the cream-and-brandy
cocktails, going about like a technician, gauging their effect
on haunch and thigh when all the time it is I who love him,
I who could have pleased him eternally if only life had
broken differently. But I am scrawny now, I am swept like
a leaf around corners, battered by the slightest wind. My
elbows rattle against my ribs and I have to spend half the
day in bed so a gram or two of what I eat will stay with me,

for if I do not, the fats and creams will vanish, burned up in my own insatiable furnace, and what little flesh I have will melt away.

Cruel as it may sound, I know where to place the blame. It was vanity, all vanity, and I hate them most for that. It was not my vanity, for I have always been a simple soul; I reconciled myself early to reenforced chairs and loose garments, to the spattering of remarks. Instead of heeding them I plugged in, and I would have been happy to let it go at that, going through life with my radio in my bodice, for while I never drew cries of admiration, no one ever blanched and turned away.

But they were vain and in their vanity my frail father, my pale, scrawny mother saw me not as an entity but a reflection on themselves. I flush with shame to remember the excuses they made for me. "She takes after May's side of the family," my father would say, denying any responsibility. "It's only baby fat," my mother would say, jabbing her elbow into my soft flank. "Nelly is big for her age." Then she would jerk furiously, pulling my voluminous smock down to cover my knees. That was when they still consented to be seen with me. In that period they would stuff me with pies and roasts before we went anywhere, filling me up so I would not gorge myself in public. Even so I had to take thirds, fourths, fifths and so I was a humiliation to them.

In time I was too much for them and they stopped taking me out; they made no more attempts to explain. Instead they tried to think of ways to make me look better; the doctors tried the fool's poor battery of pills; they tried to make me join a club. For a while my mother and I did exercises; we would sit on the floor, she in a black leotard, I in my smock. Then she would do the brisk one-two, one-two and I would make a few passes at my toes. But I had to listen, I had to plug in, and after I was plugged in naturally I had to find something to eat; Tommy might sing and I always ate when Tommy sang, and so I would leave her there on the floor, still going one-two, one-two. For a while after that they tried locking up the food. Then they began to cut into my meals.

That was the cruelest time. They would refuse me bread, they would plead and cry, plying me with lettuce and telling me it was all for my own good. My own good. Couldn't they hear my vitals crying out? I fought, I screamed, and when that failed I suffered in silent obedience until finally hunger drove me into the streets. I would lie in bed, made brave by the Monets and Barry Arkin and the Philadons coming in over the radio, and Tommy (there was never enough; I heard him a hundred times a day and it was never enough; how bitter that seems now!). I would hear them and then when my parents were asleep I would unplug and go out into the neighborhood. The first few nights I begged, throwing myself on the mercy of passers-by and then plunging into the bakery, bringing home everything I didn't eat right there in the shop. I got money quickly enough; I didn't even have to ask. Perhaps it was my bulk, perhaps it was my desperate subverbal cry of hunger; I found I had only to approach and the money was mine. As soon as they saw me, people would whirl and bolt, hurling a purse or wallet into my path as if to slow me in my pursuit; they would be gone before I could even express my thanks. Once I was shot at. Once a stone lodged itself in my flesh.

At home my parents continued with their tears and pleas. They persisted with their skim milk and their chops, ignorant of the life I lived by night. In the daytime I was complaisant, dozing between snacks, feeding on the sounds which played in my ear, coming from the radio concealed in my dress. Then, when night fell, I unplugged; it gave a certain edge to things, knowing I would not plug in again until I was ready to eat. Some nights this only meant going to one of the caches in my room, bringing forth bottles and cartons and cans. On other nights I had to go into the streets, finding money where I could. Then I would lay in a new supply of cakes and rolls and baloney from the delicatessen and several cans of ready-made frosting and perhaps a fletch of bacon or some ham; I would toss in a basket of oranges to ward off scurvy and a carton of candy bars for quick energy. Once I had enough I would go back to my room, concealing food here and there, rearranging my nest of pillows and comforters. I would open the first pie or the first half-gallon of ice cream and then, as I began, I would plug in.

You had to plug in; everybody that mattered was plugged in. It was our bond, our solace and our power, and it wasn't a matter of being distracted, or occupying time. The sound was what mattered, that and the fact that fat or thin, asleep or awake, you were important when you plugged in, and you knew that through fire and flood and adversity, through contumely and hard times there was this single bond, this common heritage; strong or weak, eternally gifted or wretched and ill-loved, we were all plugged in.

Tommy, beautiful Tommy Fango, the others paled to nothing next to him. Everybody heard him in those days; they played him two or three times an hour but you never knew when it would be so you were plugged in and listening hard every living moment; you ate, you slept, you drew breath for the moment when they would put on one of Tommy's records, you waited for his voice to fill the room. Cold cuts and cupcakes and game hens came and went during that period in my life, but one thing was constant; I always had a cream pie thawing and when they played the first bars of "When a Widow" and Tommy's voice first flexed and uncurled, I was ready, I would eat the cream pie during Tommy's midnight show. The whole world waited in those days; we waited through endless sunlight, through nights of drumbeats and monotony, we all waited for Tommy Fango's records, and we waited for that whole unbroken hour of Tommy, his midnight show. He came on live at midnight in those days; he sang, broadcasting from the Hotel Riverside, and that was beautiful, but more important, he talked, and while he was talking he made everything all right. Nobody was lonely when Tommy talked; he brought us all together on that midnight show, he talked and made us powerful, he talked and finally he sang. You have to imagine what it was like, me in the night, Tommy, the pie. In a while I would go to a place where I had to live on Tommy and only Tommy, to a time when hearing Tommy would bring back the pie, all the poor lost pies . . .

Tommy's records, his show, the pie . . . that was perhaps the happiest period of my life. I would sit and listen and I would eat and eat and eat. So great was my bliss that it became torture to put away the food at daybreak; it grew harder and harder for me to hide the cartons and the cans and the bottles, all the residue of my happiness. Perhaps a bit of bacon fell into the register; perhaps an egg rolled under the bed and began to smell. All right, perhaps I did become careless, continuing my revels into the morning, or I may have been thoughtless enough to leave a jelly roll unfinished on the rug. I became aware that they were watching, lurking just outside my door, plotting as I ate. In time they broke in on me, weeping and pleading, lamenting over every ice cream carton and crumb of pie; then they threatened. Finally they restored the food they had taken from me in the daytime, thinking to curtail my eating at night. Folly. By that time I needed it all, I shut myself in with it and would not listen. I ignored their cries of hurt pride, their outpourings of wounded vanity, their puny little threats. Even if I had listened, I could not have forestalled what happened next.

I was so happy that last day. There was a Smithfield ham, mine, and I remember a jar of cherry preserves, mine, and I remember bacon, pale and white on Italian bread. I remember sounds downstairs and before I could take warning, an assault, a company of uniformed attendants, the sting of a hypodermic gun. Then the ten of them closed in and grappled me into a sling, or net, and heaving and straining, they bore me down the stairs. I'll never forgive you, I cried, as they bundled me into the ambulance. I'll never forgive you, I bellowed as my mother in a last betrayal took away my radio, and I cried out one last time, as my father removed a hambone from my breast: I'll never forgive you. And I never have.

It is painful to describe what happened next. I remember three days of horror and agony, of being too weak, finally, to cry out or claw the walls. Then at last I was quiet and they moved me into a sunny, pastel, chintz-bedizened room. I remember that there were flowers on the dresser and someone was watching me.

"What are you in for?" she said.

I could barely speak for weakness. "Despair."

"Hell with that," she said, chewing. "You're in for food."

"What are you eating?" I tried to raise my head.

"Chewing. Inside of the mouth. It helps."

"I'm going to die."

"Everybody thinks that at first. I did." She tilted her head in an attitude of grace. "You know, this is a very exclusive school."

Her name was Ramona and as I wept silently, she filled me in. This was a last resort for the few who could afford to send their children here. They prettied it up with a schedule of therapy, exercise, massage; we would wear dainty pink smocks and talk of art and theater; from time to time we would attend classes in elocution and hygiene. Our parents would say with pride that we were away at Faircrest, an elegant finishing school; we knew better—it was a prison and we were being starved.

"It's a world I never made," said Ramona, and I knew that her parents were to blame, even as mine were. Her mother liked to take the children into hotels and casinos, wearing her thin daughters like a garland of jewels. Her father followed the sun on his private yacht, with the pennants flying and his children on the fantail, lithe and tanned. He would pat his flat, tanned belly and look at Ramona in disgust. When it was no longer possible to hide her, he gave in to blind pride. One night they came in a launch and took her away. She had been here six months now, and had lost almost a hundred pounds. She must have been monumental in her prime; she was still huge.

"We live from day to day," she said. "But you don't know the worst."

"My radio," I said in a spasm of fear. "They took away my radio."

"There is a reason," she said. "They call it therapy."

I was mumbling in my throat, in a minute I would scream.

"Wait." With ceremony, she pushed aside a picture and touched a tiny switch and then, like sweet balm for my panic, Tommy's voice flowed into the room.

When I was quiet she said, "You only hear him once a day."

"No."

"But you can hear him any time you want to. You hear him when you need him most."

But we were missing the first few bars and so we shut up and listened, and after "When a Widow" was over we sat quietly for a moment, her resigned, me weeping, and then Ramona threw another switch and the Sound filtered into the room, and it was almost like being plugged in.

"Try not to think about it."

"I'll die."

"If you think about it you *will* die. You have to learn to use it instead. In a minute they will come with lunch," Ramona said and as The Screamers sang sweet background, she went on in a monotone: "A chop. One lousy chop with a piece of lettuce and maybe some gluten bread. I pretend it's a leg of lamb, that works if you eat very, very slowly and think about Tommy the whole time; then if you look at your picture of Tommy you can turn the lettuce into anything you want, Caesar salad or a whole smorgasbord, and if you say his name over and over you can pretend a whole bombe or torte if you want to and . . ."

"I'm going to pretend a ham and kidney pie and a watermelon filled with chopped fruits and Tommy and I are in the Rainbow Room and we're going to finish up with Fudge

Royale . . ." I almost drowned in my own saliva; in the background I could almost hear Tommy and I could hear Ramona saying, "Capon, Tommy would like capon, canard à l'orange, Napoleons, tomorrow we will save Tommy for lunch and listen while we eat . . ." and I thought about that, I thought about listening and imagining whole cream pies and I went on, ". . . lemon pie, rice pudding, a whole Edam cheese . . . I think I'm going to live."

The matron came in the next morning at breakfast, and stood as she would every day, tapping red fingernails on one svelte hip, looking on in revulsion as we fell on the glass of orange juice and the hard-boiled egg. I was too weak to control myself; I heard a shrill snivelling sound and realized only from her expression that it was my own voice: "Please, just some bread, a stick of butter, anything, I could lick the dishes if you'd let me, only please don't leave me like this, please . . ." I can still see her sneer as she turned her back.

I felt Ramona's loyal hand on my shoulder. "There's always toothpaste but don't use too much at once or they'll come and take it away from you."

I was too weak to rise and so she brought it and we shared the tube and talked about all the banquets we had ever known, and when we got tired of that we talked about Tommy, and when that failed, Ramona went to the switch and we heard "When a Widow," and that helped for a while, and then we decided that tomorrow we would put off "When a Widow" until bedtime because then we would have something to look forward to all day. Then lunch came and we both wept.

It was not just hunger: after a while the stomach begins to devour itself and the few grams you toss it at mealtimes assuage it so that in time the appetite itself begins to fail. After hunger comes depression. I lay there, still too weak to get about, and in my misery I realized that they could bring me roast pork and watermelon and Boston cream pie without ceasing; they could gratify all my dreams and I would only weep helplessly, because I no longer had the strength to eat. Even then, when I thought I had reached rock bottom, I had not comprehended the worst. I noticed it first in Ramona. Watching her at the mirror, I said, in fear:

"You're thinner."

She turned with tears in her eyes. "Nelly, I'm not the only one."

I looked around at my own arms and saw that she was right: there was one less fold of flesh above the elbow; there was one less wrinkle at the wrist. I turned my face to the wall and all Ramona's talk of food and Tommy did not comfort me. In desperation she turned on Tommy's voice, but as he sang I lay back and contemplated the melting of my own flesh.

"If we stole a radio we could hear him again," Ramona said, trying to soothe me. "We could hear him when he sings tonight."

Tommy came to Faircrest on a visit two days later, for reasons that I could not then understand. All the other girls lumbered into the assembly hall to see him, thousands of pounds of agitated flesh. It was that morning that I discovered I could walk again, and I was on my feet, struggling into the pink tent in a fury to get to Tommy, when the matron intercepted me.

"Not you, Nelly."

"I have to get to Tommy. I have to hear him sing."

"Next time, maybe." With a look of naked cruelty she added, "You're a disgrace. You're still too gross."

I lunged, but it was too late; she had already shot the bolt. And so I sat in the midst of my diminishing body, suffering while every other girl in the place listened to him sing. I knew then that I had to act; I would regain myself somehow, I would find food and regain my flesh and then I would go to Tommy. I would use force if I had to, but I would hear him sing. I raged through the room all that morning, hearing the shrieks of five hundred girls, the thunder of their feet, but even when I pressed myself against the wall I could not hear Tommy's voice.

Yet Ramona, when she came back to the room, said the most interesting thing. It was some time before she could speak at all, but in her generosity she played "When a Widow" while she regained herself, and then she spoke:

"He came for something, Nelly. He came for something he didn't find."

"Tell about what he was wearing. Tell what his throat did when he sang."

"He looked at all the *before* pictures, Nelly. The matron was trying to make him look at the *afters* but he kept looking at the *befores* and shaking his head and then he found one and put it in his pocket and if he hadn't found it, he wasn't going to sing."

I could feel my spine stiffen. "Ramona, you've got to help me. I must go to him."

That night we staged a daring break. We clubbed the attendant when he brought dinner, and once we had him under the bed we ate all the chops and gluten bread on his cart and then we went down the corridor, lifting bolts, and when we were a hundred strong we locked the matron in her office and raided the dining hall, howling and eating everything we could find. I ate that night, how I ate, but even as I ate I was aware of a fatal lightness in my bones, a failure in capacity, and so they found me in the frozen food locker, weeping over a chain of link sausage, inconsolable because I understood that they had spoiled it for me, they with their chops and their gluten bread; I could never eat as I once had, I would never be myself again.

In my fury I went after the matron with a ham hock, and when I had them all at bay I took a loin of pork for sustenance and I broke out of that place. I had to get to Tommy before I got any thinner; I had to try. Outside the gate I stopped a car and hit the driver with the loin of pork and then I drove to the Hotel Riverside, where Tommy always stayed. I made my way up the fire stairs on little cat feet and when the valet went to his suite with one of his velveteen suits I followed, quick as a tigress, and the next moment I was inside. When all was quiet I tiptoed to his door and stepped inside.

He was magnificent. He stood at the window, gaunt and beautiful; his blond hair fell to his waist and his shoulders shriveled under a heartbreaking double-breasted pea-green velvet suit. He did not see me at first; I drank in his image and then, delicately, cleared my throat. In the second that he turned and saw me, everything seemed possible.

"It's you." His voice throbbed.

"I had to come."

Our eyes fused and in that moment I believed that we two could meet, burning as a single, lambent flame, but in the next second his face had crumpled in disappointment; he brought a picture from his pocket, a fingered, cracked photograph, and he looked from it to me and back at the photograph, saying, "My darling, you've fallen off."

"Maybe it's not too late," I cried, but we both knew I would fail.

And fail I did, even though I ate for days, for five desperate, heroic weeks; I threw pies into the breach, fresh hams and whole sides of beef, but those sad days at the food farm, the starvation and the drugs have so upset my chemistry that it cannot be restored; no matter what I eat I fall off and I continue to fall off; my body is a halfway house for foods I can no longer assimilate. Tommy watches, and because he knows he almost had me, huge and round and beautiful, Tommy mourns. He eats less and less now. He eats like a bird and lately he has refused to sing; strangely, his records have begun to disappear.

And so a whole nation waits.

"I almost had her," he says, when they beg him to resume his midnight shows; he will not sing, he won't talk, but his hands describe the mountain of woman he has longed for all his life.

And so I have lost Tommy, and he has lost me, but I am doing my best to make it up to him. I own Faircrest now, and in the place where Ramona and I once suffered I use my skills on the girls Tommy wants me to cultivate. I can put twenty pounds on a girl in a couple of weeks and I don't mean bloat, I mean solid fat. Ramona and I feed them up and once a week we weigh and I poke the upper arm with a special stick and I will not be satisfied until the stick goes in and does not rebound because all resiliency is gone. Each week I bring out my best and Tommy shakes his head in misery because the best is not yet good enough, none of them are what I once was. But one day the time and the girl will be right—would that it were me—the time and the girl will be right and Tommy will sing again. In the meantime, the whole world waits; in the meantime, in a private wing well away from the others, I keep my special cases; the matron, who grows fatter as I watch her. And Mom. And Dad.

FAT CITY

by *Burr Snider*

Froggie is the official door person, the greeter of guests. Every time a new group of revellers arrives froggie flops across the floor on her kerploppy splayed feet to welcome them. "Riiiivettt," she croaks in marvelous basso frog talk by way of greeting and digs their reaction to being ushered in by a frog. That's a sensational costume froggie has on; you can bet it's no Woolworth's number. That's one frog suit that cost some bucks. There's the bell again and there goes froggie now. Uh-oh, there's a new guy, a stranger in this party just arriving, he doesn't know a soul here. Watch this.

Froggie ignores the rest of the newcomers and attaches herself to the strange guy. She's so short she only reaches up to about the middle of his chest, short and exceedingly rotund. "Flies?" she murmurs, beginning to nibble around the guy's chest with her thick, enormously exaggerated froggie lips. "Any flies? . . . Looking for flies. . . ." Nibble nibble. The guy is backed up against the wall trying to recall if anything in his experience up to now has prepared him for handling a rapacious frog socially, but he's drawing a blank.

"A-*ha!*" exclaims froggie suddenly, jumping back in mock amazement and pointing a finger triumphantly. "At last a fly!" she shouts, rolling her great froggie head in dizzy anticipation. Pouncing again she nibbles voraciously. Cackles of laughter erupt from the other party-ers. The guy himself is plastered rigidly against the wall; his uncertain smile glitters like a cheap rhinestone appliqué. Froggie won't let go. He manages a nervous laugh: how far is this going to go? Not much farther, thank God. Another gaggle of arrivals has just come in and froggie's attention is reluctantly diverted. Whew!

Great party! It's being held in one of those Southern suburban dwelling complexes which aspire to the manor manner. It's Halloween and all the makings of seasonal festivity are abundantly present, indeed the groaning board seems actually to sag under the weight of the holiday victuals. Lambent loops of black and orange crepe paper droop from overhead, paper skeletons and goblins dangle about on strings, and from the corners comes the glow of the jack-o'-lanterns. Drinks, smokes, food, laughter, camaraderie, the blossoming of casual party lust. . . . Ya-hoo! *Great* party!

But . . . ummm, there is something . . . untoward here. Look around. There seems to be this preponderance of . . . well, this might sound unkind, but for example look over there on that couch, those three people sitting there, a guy and two chicks. I mean that's a normal-sized couch isn't it? But look how jammed in they are. There's barely room for the three of them. It looks like they're sitting on play furniture. Jesus, they're really enormous! Oh, *now* look. One of 'em is trying to get up. Oh God, poor thing. She looks like a turtle that's been flipped over on its back. *Epic* struggle. That couch is really too low. She'll never . . . yes! Terrific second effort! She's got her massive legs planted on the floor for leverage, and her short, puffy arms, looking like connected links of some balloony pop-art sausage, are vainly trying to push off from the couch, trembling madly with the effort, but the immutable force of all that massed inertia is again sucking her right back down into the cushions. Her face is twisted into doughy rolls of naked agony. . . . Ah, but now there is help. Hands cup around her elbows and, aided by a little push from the lady seated next to her, she is heaved to her feet. "Sssssshhhhhuuuuu!" she wheezes in relief, pulling herself back together. She smiles and nods gratefully to the gallants who have come to her rescue and chugs over to the buffet table.

That's it, of course. That lady has got to tip the Toledos at somewhere in the neighborhood of two-eighty, three hundred pounds, a *big* mama, and she doesn't even look out of place here! Put her down in your average crowd and she'd neon out as a monument to corpulence, but here she's just folks! Isn't this wild?

"Isn't this wild?" The new guy, the stranger that froggie worked over, has gotten separated from his friends, and he's just been sort of slinking about taking all this in. This chick has been noticing his openmouthed wonderment, chuckling as she watched the amazement race over his face, and she's just joined him at his vantage point in the hallway. She's not what you'd call petite herself, this lady isn't, but in comparison to most here she looks downright svelte. "Isn't this *wild?*" she's asking the guy. "Have you ever seen more oof on the hoof in one place in your life? These are all ricers, in case you didn't know. Damn near everyone here is on the rice diet, or has been on it."

Now it dawns on him. The *rice* diet. Of course. We're in Durham. Duke University, sure. This is the thing, what's his name, Buddy Hackett, is always boosting on the talk shows. Kempner is the guy's name. Dr. Kempner's rice diet. Ask you a question, he says to the girl. If all these people are on this diet, which I know not a thing about except it is said to be a very tough regimen, what about the old groaning board over there and all those pudgy folks gathered around it? What about those people sitting over there bent over those paper plates heaped so copiously with the potato salad and the cold cuts and that gorgeous orange-and-black-dyed bread? What about those big platters laden with brownies and chocolate-chip cookies, and listen, what about that lady back in the bedroom who is huddled over a plate of food that I have rarely seen the likes of, so intent on getting the most in the quickest that she is shoving great pawfuls into her maw, hand over hand? What about that?

"Ah, but they're cheating," says the lady. "Look at them. Look how guilty they look, how they won't meet your eye. They know what they're doing to themselves. They're paying big money to come here and starve off pounds on the rice diet, and they're throwing it all away like there's no tomorrow. Listen, I can empathize with them. They're starving. I doubt if you've ever been as hungry as most of these people are. Some of them are sick with hunger. I've been driven to cheating like this myself before. Look at me, I ask you. The only difference is I don't have the guts or the balls or whatever to do it where everybody can see me."

The lady laughs. "It's a good thing Kempner's in Europe, though. Probably most of these people wouldn't be doing this out in the open if he was here. They're scared to death of him. They say that he can look at your urine specimen and tell exactly what you have been eating."

Of course, the lady points out, as you can see not everybody here is fat. But just about everybody here is freaky in some way, that she'll guarantee. "The ricers attract all the local flakos."

Back in the bedroom things have gotten stoned slapstick. The very pudgy girl is still at it, her hands like dual metronomes slugging away at that grub. "Jesus, lookit her!" whoops another lady. "She can't get it in fast enough. Here, oinkie, lemme help ya." She grabs a big handful of the potato salad and smears it onto the other girl's mouth, trying to stuff it down her throat. "Mmmmmmmmph!" sputters the hungry girl, shaking her head in an attempt to resist the other's hand. But her helper is not to be denied. Another handful, most of which ends up on the bed. "That's right, grunt-grunt, stuff it on in there. It's only costing you about forty dollars a bite," she roars. Now they both have potato salad smeared all over themselves. The smearee is trying helplessly to suppress her giggles, but finally it spews out, laughter, food and everything all over her friend, and they collapse in a paroxysm of uncontrolled hilarity in each other's arms onto the bed.

The room is in an uproar. Another of the portly ladies jumps up and pirouettes her ungainly bulk around the room, running her hands up and down her Mother Earth corpus in a slinky self-parody. "Here it is, folks," she blusters, carny-style. "The five-thousand-dollar figure. That's right. Five big ones. Several months of rice and five thousand dollars and you can have a shape just like mine. Now if you folks would care to step in a little closer. . . ."

"Do you want to know who the most exploited person in the world is? The fat man, the fat person. Fat people are almost an ethnic group, but one that nobody has any qualms about doing a job on. You never hear on radio and TV anymore any jokes about spades or Jews or P.R.'s, but the fat man gets it from everybody. Ha-ha, the jolly fat man. Give us a yuk, fat man. Make us howl, fat lady.

"Do you have any idea what it's like to be made aware every day of your life that you're a freak? I'm not talking about the strangers on the street who stare at you and point you out to their kids right there where you can see them. I mean from your own family, the people who are supposed to love you. I think it usually starts at about age ten, for some people maybe earlier, but, yeah, for most it's about ten. See that's just about when your parents realize that this isn't just baby fat that Junior or Sis is carrying around, it's not going to magically fall away someday to reveal the little darling they've been waiting for. Yeah, about ten. From then on you are made aware of every bite of food you put in your mouth. You ask any obese person, I bet every one of them will tell you that for most of their lives they never put a bite in their mouth that they didn't feel guilty about, at least way down deep. That's a lot of accumulated guilt that fat people carry around with them.

"So say you're ten years old and Mom and Dad realize they got this chubby little monster on their hands. They don't know how to handle it so they start making the rounds of the doctors. They put you on diets and then they harp at you so about not cheating that you cheat just out of nervousness. Lots of times the parents are big eaters themselves, you know, and that makes it even tougher. Like in a lot of Jewish families homelife is still more or less centered around the table and you get the old Yiddishe

Mama thing. Eat, eat, I'm up all night cooking you shouldn't eat? Except for you, fatty, you don't eat. Keep your hands off the mashed potatoes.

"Who knows why you're fat in the first place? Maybe it is because your body requires less or something. But you're just as hungry. Or sometimes you know your parents are into their own thing and you're just not getting enough attention from them. So you tap them on the shoulder and you say, 'Hey, look at me. I'm fat.' Sure, it's negative attention you're getting, but if you're feeling left out you'll be glad to take any kind of attention you can get.

"In school your distinction is that you're the fat kid in the class. No matter what else you do. You got two choices: you either clam up and go inside yourself, live a fantasy life—and most of the fantasy is about all this fat suddenly, miraculously, dropping off of you—or you become super outgoing. You become the happy fat kid. Well, like the paper boy said, I got news for you. There's no such thing as a happy fat kid."

Gordon (the names are changed but the voices are true) is just about as likable a guy as you ever want to meet. He's smart and quick and funny and perceptive, and possessed of an appealing sort of abashed charm that is guaranteed to win you over. Gordon tips in at something around 350 pounds. At five feet nine this girth gives him the shape of a droopy double pyramid, the bases of which are joined together at his waist. When his arms are at rest they hang at a forty-five-degree angle from the vertical, pushed out by the outward slopes of his upper body. To say that Gordon is fat would not be hitting the note. For him, and for many ricers, the word needs some baroqueing up; needs some plump and squiggly little curlicues to lend it the requisite, ah, avoirdupois. Still it is possible to see handsomeness lurking like a sneak thief down there beneath the billows. Maybe if Gordon were still up around 511, which he has reached on occasion, all that would be totally obscured, but now a wisp of the promise remains. Like so many fat people, once you exhibit a genuine interest, Gordon is so disarmingly open about his obesity, its roots and ramifications, that you begin to marvel at his unsparing honesty. But he's been thinking about these things for a long time. As he says, it's hard for him to kid himself anymore. "When you're fat that's all you ever think about, so you get pretty contemptuous of the tricks you can play on yourself." Gordon is a believer in what he calls the "invalid theory" of obesity, which can be summed up in this one phrase: "Don't bother me, I can't cope. I'm too fat."

"See, when you're fat you don't have to take responsibility for anything but your fatness. You don't have to go out and meet people and you don't have to take the chance of getting hurt that contact always poses. You can just stay in the dark and brood and fester. Nobody is particularly going to take the trouble to try to get to know a fat person. So the fat is nice protection if you look at it that way. It's literally a nice thick wall insulating you from contact."

Gordon's been coming to Durham for twelve years now. Sometimes he stays here even when he's not "on service" with the Kempner program: "I guess I like it here. I feel comfortable and accepted here. Even most of the townies are used to the ricers so they don't turn and stare at you in the street when you walk past. They just assume you're on the diet. Sometimes one of the grits [townspeople] will ask me something that shows he just assumes I'm a ricer, like how's things on the diet? I look at him like he's crazy and I say, What kind of diet? I don't know from diets. I'm jut passing through here on my way to Florida."

For him the rice diet has been only intermittently successful. He has achieved some quite dramatic weight losses, most notably a 230-pound drop in a fourteen-month period in 1967-68 (he says he was inspired by a girl he was in love with at the time), but every time the pounds came piling back. "The last significant weight loss I had, what would be significant to you, was eighty pounds. But it was nothing to me. I hardly looked any different."

Gordon doesn't make any pretensions to an aesthetic love of food. "I'm a junkie," he says, "not a gourmet. When

I go on a binge it's usually snackies, whatever's quickest and easiest, lots of TV dinners. Some say if you ingest ten times your body weight in calories you maintain without gaining. Like I weigh 350, so I could eat 3500 calories a day. Well, one stinking TV dinner has 500 calories in it and I can inhale *three* of them without blinking. Right now I'm not dieting. I guess I just don't have any incentive. But that doesn't mean I don't feel guilty when I go overboard. Last night's an example. I'm driving home and I know I'm gonna have trouble getting past Ken's Quickie Mart which stays open late. My goddamned car just follows its nose right into the parking lot. I picked up an eight-inch frozen pizza, eight ounces of American cheese, some apples and a handful of Mounds candy bars. Just for a snack. Burnt the goddamned pizza so bad I couldn't eat it. Pissed me off 'cause by that time Ken's was closed and I was really hungry. And this was all after dinner, mind you. For dinner I had had shrimp cocktail and prime ribs, the works.

"Oh, I'll tell you something else crazy about this town. I never saw anything like it. Everywhere you go, I mean *everywhere,* they got these sandwiches for sale. You know what I'm talking about? In cellophane wrappers? Like ham and cheese and tuna and egg salad. Chicken salad, like that. Everywhere. At gas stations, in the movies. I went into a tailor's the other day and there was a pile of those rotten sandwiches on the counter. You can wolf down a couple while you're waiting for your dry cleaning, for Christ's sake.

"I'm from New York, you know, and somehow Durham cheating and New York cheating are different. Here, like I said, I don't mind going out all that much because these people are used to us. But in New York you really stand out, you know, so you try to stay in as much as possible. Which isn't hard really 'cause it's so easy to order out. I must be the best customer that Rocky Lee's pizza ever had. I once had this fantasy that the delivery trucks from Rocky Lee's and Jay Tang's Chinese restaurant and The Steak Joint had this enormous wreck on the corner of Sixty-fourth Street and First Avenue. I thought, Jesus, what a great head start on a diet if those trucks were just put out of commission for a week."

"It is not a new experience that special diets are burdensome and require the faithful cooperation of physician and patient. The rice-fruit-sugar diet is certainly no exception."—"Compensation of Renal Metabolic Dysfunction: Treatment of Kidney Disease and Hypertensive Vascular Disease with Rice Diet," by Dr. Walter Kempner. *North Carolina Medical Journal,* February, 1945.

Recognition didn't come easy for Dr. Kempner, God knows. When he first started pushing his rice diet back in the early Forties he was met with a pretty big ration of ridicule from the medical establishment. It was only to be expected. After all, he was turning accepted dietary rules upside down. For years he had been studying the metabolism of deranged cells, first in his native Germany, and then, after Hitler's accession, here in the States at Duke. His interest was focused on the effects of diet on people suffering from vascular and renal diseases—diseases such as nephritis and nephrosis (deadly kidney ailments), high blood pressure, heart disease and diabetes. Through his research Kempner became convinced that diet played a much larger role in the incidence of such diseases than was believed at the time. Salt, he concluded, was the major poisoner. What was needed was a regimen which would be salt free, which contained a minimum of protein and fat (and, of course, cholesterol), and which would maintain a balance of essential amino acids and certain chemical substances called "electrolytes" in the body. He was struck by the fact that in geographical areas where rice was a primary diet staple, the Far East, for example, the incidence of these diseases was demonstrably less frequent than in Western countries where comparatively little rice—but proportionately more fat—was consumed. Eureka. After some tinkering around he found that a severely restricted regimen consisting of rice, fruit and fruit juices—supplemented with vitamins—met the requirements best. The fact that that diet was high in carbohydrates and low in protein didn't sit too well with nutrition experts of the day, and many dismissed Kempner as just another faddist. He himself at first didn't think such a stringent program could be maintained by a patient for sustained periods, until a lucky accident convinced him otherwise. In 1942 he had started a patient, a middle-aged North Carolina farm wife suffering from chronic nephritis and an enlarged heart, on the diet, instructing her to return to the clinic at the end of two weeks. But she misunderstood his German accent and didn't return for two months, her condition remarkably improved. Kempner was soon able to produce convincing documented evidence proving the efficacy of his diet—that not only was it capable of arresting the progress of the diseases being treated, but in some cases, if followed closely over a long-enough period, it was actually effecting repairs in what had heretofore been thought of as terminal diseases. More and more doctors began referring their chronic kidney, hypertension and diabetic cases to Kempner's clinic.

"There are plenty of people walking around today who are alive because of the Kempner diet," says Mary Wolfe, a slim and gracious and quite healthy-looking lady who appears to be in her early fifties. "I know because I'm one of them." Mary lives in Durham now, in a beautifully restored cabin outside town. She came to love the area through her frequent visits to Durham over the years, and now, although there is no real reason for her to be near the clinic, she prefers to stay.

"I suffered from hypertension and it looked for a while as if I would die. Doctor after doctor could do nothing for me. Finally I had a sympathectomy, which at that time, in the Forties, was considered quite a last-ditch operation. When it didn't seem to have done any good, a doctor recommended that I come to Durham and try the rice diet. I did, and slowly began to improve. I lived on rice and fruit for a long time but eventually it was liberalized so I could have other things, vegetables and even a little meat, but never any salt. And here I am now, all these years later, feeling very well, thank you."

Mary feels that Kempner has never really gotten the kind of recognition that he deserves. "He took on people that nobody else could help. I remember children dying of terminal kidney diseases. He put them on the diet and watched them closely and some of them actually improved. He was able to add months, and sometimes years, to their lives after they had been given up for dead."

Gradually resistance to the revolutionary new diet died away, ever so gradually as it were, as Kempner and his colleagues built up an impressive file of successful cases. In the early years of the diet it had been noticed of course that a significant weight loss usually occurred in those who undertook the regimen, and eventually Kempner began accepting patients whose only apparent problem was obesity—as opposed to the vascular and renal patients. It was and is, however, Kempner's contention that there is no such thing as "just" obesity. He feels that the chronically overweight condition is invariably accompanied by attendant problems, that obesity frequently is a sign that the body has been damaged. For this reason he subjects everyone going on the diet to a probing comprehensive battery of tests and consultation before their weight-loss regimen begins.

Over the years more and more obesity patients were accepted at the clinic, but it was in 1952 that a marked increase was noted. Then in 1968 Mrs. Betty Hughes, whose husband was the governor of New Jersey at the time, wrote a highly laudatory article in *Ladies' Home Journal* about her successful weight loss on the diet and soon after that most of Kempner's patients had obesity problems.

"Things were a lot different when I first came down here sixteen years ago," says Elaine, who at 230 pounds, even though she is down a hundred from a year ago, is not one of the rice diet's most successful examples. "I was an obesity case in 1958," she continues. "I was seventeen

years old. I weighed 268 pounds. Many of the other patients were here for hypertension and kidney trouble and
stuff, terminal diseases mostly. It was pretty horrible. The
clinic had outgrown the hospital where they used to keep
all the patients, and they had just set up the rice houses—
one on Lamond Street and one on Mangum—where everybody lived and ate. I was surrounded by death. In those
days they had time to look after you and I was watched like
a hawk. Now there are too many patients for that and things
are a little looser." Elaine dropped a hundred pounds that
first time around and went back north to finish school. But
in a year's time she had gained it all back and then some
and was back in Durham. She figures she's spent almost
half of the intervening years here and has been on the
program at least fifteen times.

"When I first used to come down here I was really a
hateful kid. I would throw tantrums and scream and do
anything for attention. The nurses despised me. One time
Kempner caught me cheating and he put me in the hospital
for a supervised fast. I had nothing but distilled water for
twenty-eight days. He knew I was into psychology in school
so he told me I should study the psychological effects of
starvation. By the end of the fast I had lost thirty pounds.

"Later that same year I got sick and got down to 161.
Kempner wanted me to go to 145 and a battle of wills
began. I left the hospital at 132. I shot back up to 150 in
two weeks' time. I used to volunteer to help the nurses with
the food trays so I could steal off them."

Elaine's all-time high was 411 pounds. She has a picture
of herself at that weight taped to the refrigerator door in
her apartment. Last year when she returned to Durham
after an absence of several years she was so heavy that her
legs couldn't support her and one of her knees had given
out. She had to use a cane to walk. "You run into a lot of
bizarre things in an atmosphere like this one," she laughs.
"A lot of humor here, although most of it is pretty desperate humor. You know like most ricers are scared to death

of Kempner. People will do anything not to incur his wrath. There's a weigh-in every morning at the rice houses too, so if there are any suspicious jumps in weight you can count on getting some crap from the staff. But there's always a way to beat it. People will go out on a binge and then take these enormous doses of laxative and void it all. Or you can take diuretics too. 'Course they dehydrate you and make you lose abnormal amounts of potassium. People get very sick on them but they go right back out and do them again.

"You know, my whole life revolves around being fat. It gets to be this very vicious circle. I'll start to feel guilty about doing this to myself and that will bring on stress which makes me nervous, so I begin to eat, which brings on more guilt. Finally you just say, What the hell, I'm a rotten son of a bitch anyway, and you just eat some more. It's like a trap you can't get out of. But after all this, after years of going through this kind of self-hate and loneliness and unhappiness, of always getting hurt because of the supersensitivity you build up, I'm not ready to throw the towel in. I'm still working at it in my fashion. I guess that says something."

Jeannie is just now experiencing what must be quite a delightful sensation: she is discovering for the first time in her life that she's attractive. Jeannie's dropped more than a hundred pounds in the eleven months or so that she's been in Durham and although she's still a touch pudgy at 147—twenty pounds over her goal—there is almost no resemblance between the present Jeannie and the bloated blob that stares dully out at you in her "before" picture. Jeannie is a tough, funny girl in her early thirties, and she is fond of shrewd observations about fat life-styles.

"You're gonna be seeing a lot of 'before' pictures in Durham," she says, laughing. "Anytime anybody is successful on a diet the first thing they do when they meet you is to find some excuse to whip out the old 'before' picture. I guess you can understand why. I look at old pictures of me and I can't believe it myself. I don't think fat people really know what they look like. They avoid seeing themselves. And you have no idea what a trip it is to find out that you really have a face, with definition and all. You know there are a lot of things that most women take for granted that just don't happen to a fat chick. Like guys are just now beginning to do nice, polite things for me, lighting my cigarette and opening doors for me. Nobody does that kind of thing for a fat woman. It's really heavenly."

Jeannie's been going on—and falling off—diets ever since she can remember. The pattern is always the same: big losses at first which dwindle down until you hit a plateau that you can't seem to get past. Then you get discouraged and start cheating. "I've tried 'em all, baby." She laughs. "You gotta figure that by the time someone comes here for the rice diet they've already tried every goddamned method in the world for losing weight. Counting calories, counting carbohydrates, eating only one thing for weeks, water diets, hospital fasts, sleep cures, every kind of fad diet you can imagine out of the women's magazines, Metrecal, uppers, downers, injections . . . do you know there's one where they inject you with the urine of a pregnant woman and it supposedly makes you lose weight? But I'm married to a guy who eats all day and never gains an ounce. So all I do is cook. What am I supposed to do? For me coming to Durham was really the last gasp. I mean it's a pretty major move. You give up your home and your family, if you're a guy you got to take all this time away from your job or your business, and you move down here for months, in some cases for years, just to lose weight. You got to be pretty desperate to put yourself through that."

Jeannie stayed on the rice diet for six months, but when she stopped losing weight she switched over to still another diet program administered by Dr. Richard Stuelke under the auspices of the Duke Student Health Program. Jeannie's case more or less defines the coordinates of a controversy that is raging in Durham at the moment; it might be figuratively described as Kempner in this corner and Stuelke in this. Many ricers, in fact, are making the move away from the rice diet over to the Stuelke plan, which is a more relaxed and liberal regimen than Kempner allows. Buddy Hackett, who for years was one of Kempner's biggest boosters, talking up the rice diet on Carson's show, tried out Stuelke's regimen recently for a one-month period. He still has only the best of things to say about Kempner and doesn't want to get involved in the controversy. Buddy just drops into town several times a year to shed whatever excess that high living has piled on him and just as quietly he slips out.

"I lost a lot of weight on the rice diet, but I got really sick on it," says Jeannie. "I was always feeling dizzy and woozy and then I started passing out. I had my period for two months straight. When it started to look like I wasn't gonna lose any more weight I said to myself, Who needs this aggravation? and I switched over.

"See, Stuelke's diet is salt-poor in contrast to the rice diet which is salt-free. This gives him a lot more latitude in designing menus and you get to eat of lot of things Kempner forbids. As far as I'm concerned it's just about impossible to try to maintain the rice diet in normal life, even though it too loosens up some after the first few weeks. I'm not really knocking Kempner on this point—if you have a lot of weight to lose and want to do it the fastest way, his diet is probably the best—but I think Stuelke provides a nice sort of halfway house for people who want to get back to their regular lives. Also some people just can't or won't stick to the rice diet and this one is much easier. And there's another thing. Stuelke's overweight himself, and he's been even fatter than he is now, so he can empathize with you; he knows what you're going through. Kempner is like a piece of wire. He refuses to sympathize or try to identify with the patients. He's very cold and very impersonal.

"I guess you have to remember that he's been dealing

with these fat people for a long time. He probably knows more about it than anybody, so there's sure to be a method in his madness. Most people come here *wanting* to be punished for this horrible thing they've done to themselves. They're really masochistic. I think they'd eat garbage if he gave it to them. You got to remember that people who come here are very self-indulgent people, most of them pretty rich. And they've let themselves get so helpless. You see people coming in here so heavy they have to have walkers just to get around. I'm talking about four and five hundred pounds and more. I'm talking about *fat.*"

Melody is another girl who, like Jeannie, is emerging from a lifelong chrysalis of fatty tissue, only twenty or thirty pounds away from true beauty. And, like Jeannie, she is also a convert to Stuelke after half a year or so on the rice diet. She has her own reasons. "Don't let anyone kid you, all this about glandular problems and all is just crap. Maybe some people's bodies assimilate food better than others, but it still all comes down to eating too much. Even so, though, there's got to be some psychological reason *why* you do, and I think these problems ought to be attacked. But Kempner discourages you from seeing a shrink when you are on service. Nobody denies that Kempner can give you a slim body but he leaves you with a fat head. On Stuelke you can get group therapy. He encourages it.

"If you want to know what I think, though, I think a lot of ricers come back here because they like it here. You know, for the first time in your life you're surrounded by people who have the same problem you do. You find out you're not as abnormal as you thought. It's kinda comforting. Plus you gotta remember that most of the people here are not exactly playing with a full deck. This is kind of an escape into unreality for them. Funny, when you first get down here you really feel horrible. Here you are in this strange little Southern town, you've been pushed around like a goddamned cow through a few days of testing, then you go over to one of the rice houses where they feed you this thimbleful of crappy rice, and all you see are these tremendously fat people. Your first reaction is to stay aloof. You look at these . . . grotesque, overweight slobs and you think, I'm not one of those. I don't look like that. And even if I do, I'm not *really* a fat person. The *real* me, down underneath all this, is skinny. This fat is just something that happened to me. So you shy away from contact. But then after a while you begin to realize that everybody here is in the same boat, we've all got the same problems. Maybe the reasons we're fat aren't the same, but the result is. That's one of the things about obesity, it's right out there for everyone to see. Maybe we're not really any more screwed up than anyone else, but everyone can see our hang-ups. Anyway, after you get over that initial standoffishness you begin to develop some very deep relationships. There are a lot of jokes about the hanky-panky that goes on among the ricers, but I think it's this feeling of being in sort of a ghetto that causes it. You know, we're all pariahs together. Another ricer is the only one who can ever really know what you go through. Plus there's this crazy thing that seems to happen to just about everybody. When the fat starts dropping off, the old sex drive starts to come back. What it is, I think, is that fat masks feelings. When you're fat you don't want any emotional contact with anybody, you just want to be left alone. You're unfeeling and it seems like you just forget about sex. But when you start to recognize yourself again, when you start to get the feeling that maybe there's something there to like again, Jesus, you really start getting horny. Of course you need a lot of reinforcement to stick to the diet. You need some kind of *proof* that this torture you're putting yourself through—and believe me, it's pure hell—is worthwhile. What better way is there than to have somebody show some interest in you?"

Passing the day in Fat City: At the Downtowner and the Durham Hotel. At the Duke Motor Lodge. At the Cavalier

Inn (where Buddy stops when he's in town), and the Holiday Inn and the Hilton. In drab efficiencies off Gregson and combination studios on Chapel Hill Road. In the sorority-chapter ambience of the rice houses on Lamond and Mangum, the ricers morbidly molt away the days in their transient chambers, while the pounds drop off slowly, agonizingly, imperceptibly, choking back screams of deprivation, gnawing on reddened knuckles as the walls resound with the crunches, slurps, gurgles and grunts, the resplendency of remembered repasts, gargantuan grub-ups of the fantasy, aromatic juices of the imagination sending maddening wafts through the nostrils of memory, visions of: sugarplums? Sure, and what of thick, mayo-dripping B.L.T.s and triple-decker clubs impaled with those little fancy-dan toothpicks? What of good roadside greasyburgers buttressed with slices of soggy onions and puckery, acidic pickles, with sides of yummy fries swimming in viscous pools of watery catsup . . . mmm . . . marbled K.C. strips heaped in mounds upon platters, baskets of hot garlic bread with chives, bursting Idahoes all gooey with sour cream and bacon bits and gobs of butter, barbecued chips, Fritos, Twinkies, onion dip, jalapeño bean sauce, guacamole . . . veal parmigiana . . . Sara Lee, vile temptress . . . oh, those little dime pies in wax paper, little two-bite pies, ah God, Reese's peanut-butter cups, Nestle's Crunch, sludgy sundaes of axle-grease chocolate and maraschino in counterpoint . . . Jesus, stop it now, just stop it. It always starts this way, with these reveries. Just get your mind off it, don't think about it. You *know* once you start. . . . It's just crazy. You got too much into this to start cheating now, much too much. Right off the bat there was that five- or six-hundred-dollar pop for tests and consultation. Two days of being pushed and poked at and drained . . . and then that consultation with Herr Doktor. Hello, wat's you name, don' chead, be sure and wear your nametag, goodbye. Then up to a hundred and fifty a week for treatment, plus, *plus* thirty for what they call food. Forget about motel or apartment rental, away-from-home living expenses and like that. No, babe, no cheating, not when you're pumping close to a grand a month into this. Besides, whatever you eat is gonna show up in the urinalysis anyway, am I right? Aha, look! A cheeseburger! A small pizza! With anchovies! And one, two, three . . . eight. Eight Hershey's Candy Kisses! You've been cheading, are-en't you ashamed? You are a cheader. Herr Professor Doktor Kempner can read your peepee like it's an autobiography. So just forget it. Try a book. Let's see, a little Thomas Wolfe? Local boy wasn't he, from Asheville or somewhere? . . . Oh no! Not with those scrumptious descriptive passages about the feasts Mama Gant used to whip up for the boarders. And God, do you remember that one about going out to the circus early in the morning with his brother to work for free passes? Sneaking into the food tent to watch the performers shovel down those mammoth breakfasts? Do you remember how he goes on about the smell of the coffee bubbling pungently in the big silvered urns, the oatmeal and rich heavy cream, mounds of hotcakes soaking up butter and syrup, the snapping of the eggs on the grill and the rashers of smoked bacon? . . . No! And stay away from Henry Miller, too, that bastard, with his midnight sensualist's snacks of wursts and funky cheeses and Westphalian ham and moist black bread spread with sweet butter. Him with his fruits and tortes and chilled Moselles. . . .

Well, try the tube then. No cooking shows, no Julia or the Galloper, for God's sake, and just try to ignore the commercials. Ooooh, that one where they show how that butterball turkey bastes itself from the *inside* with pure butter . . . Betty Crocker . . . Pop Tarts . . . A&P . . . oooh. Take a walk. Go over to the "Y" for some volleyball. But no picking off the room-service trays on your way, so embarrassing when you get nabbed. And stay away from that poisonous little carry-out near Lamond. Dinner's only an hour away. Dinner? Some lousy super-scrubbed rice and a little fruit, glass of lousy tea? You call that dinner? And still eighty-five pounds till goal? Oh, I think I wanna die. . . .

"Lord, these folks is o-*beast!*" a local cabbie drawls in wonderment, and he ain't wrong, he ain't wrong. Most Durhamites are pretty blasé about the ricers by now (it takes a really extraordinary case to make heads swing in the street anymore), but due to the insularity of the ricers and the natural suspicions of many small-town folks, the camps coexist pretty much in an atmosphere of latent hostility. Of course the fact that most ricers don't hit town exactly penniless hasn't escaped the attention of the locals, neither the businessmen nor the Main Street cowpokes who make the easy rounds of the ricer ladies. The general sentiment of the transient diet community is probably best summed up in this quote from "The Rotund Ricer," a nonofficial, unauthorized underground sheet which mysteriously appears from time to time and whose editorial content is mostly devoted to gossip, jabs at Kempner, and a running stream of invective aimed at the locals: "Ricers are, more often than not, misunderstood, misinterpreted, misconstrued, and generally abused by almost every straight group and individual in the goddamn, half-assed city of Durham, North Carolina. We are only tolerated because we spend a goddamned lot of money in this god forsakened [sic] place. So go on and do your damnedest Durham. We can take it. And we'll leave tons of blubber all over this miserable, scroungy town."

On the other hand many of the locals resent what they consider a condescending attitude on the part of the ricers. "These people been coming here for years from places like New York and Philadelphia and Chicago, thinking that we all walk around with straw hanging out of our mouths," says a young Durham guy. "But you know something? We got some slicks of our own around here and sometimes they get that hayseed impression changed for them real fast."

To that, many ricers would say a simple "Amen."

"There's two kinds of prices in this town," says a disenchanted ricer lady from Miami. "Regular and ricer. We're the original ones you can see coming from a mile away." But these aren't necessarily unanimous views. Some ricers escape the psychic walls that dieting builds and carve out a life of their own here. Elaine, for example, is almost a local herself, she's been here so much. She has a local circle of friends, teaches in a school for abnormal children ("I think I got some special insights that can help them") and stays here much of the time even when she isn't on service.

Still, the hands across the water are few. "You want to hear something that'll really kill you?" asks Jeannie. "There's a shop here, a clothing shop, that caters to ricer women. Extra-large sizes you know? It's like one of those places where you can go and get a size-52 bathing suit if you need it, things like that. Well, you want to hear what the name of that shop is? 'The Wee Shop.' 'The *Wee* Shop!' That knocks me out. One time I asked the woman why in the world she ever decided to call the place 'The Wee Shop.' She said she thought it was kind of a cute name."

If you stay in Durham long enough you are bound to hear about Betty's Turkey Caper. Just as soldiers dig sitting around and rapping what they call war stories—tales of sexual derring-do—so ricers love swapping fables of prodigious eating feats, of super-conspicuous consumption. You hear of Jimmy G. who could knock off forty-five hot dogs in a sitting, or Ramon who can go through a case of beer in a snap, or of the unnamed guy who, after a successful stay at the clinic during which he dropped a good eighty pounds, gained twenty-one back during the car trip home by hitting every diner, general store and restaurant on the way. You talk to a lady who claims to have perfected the art of using a lettuce leaf for a mayonnaise knife when she sneaks downstairs for a midnight cheat because she knows her husband and kids have ears which are attuned to the sound of the silver drawer being opened.

But the undisputed supreme all-time number-one champion is Betty and her Turkey Caper. It comes up almost every time ricers gather. Betty wears her laurels with consummate grace and her infamy has not turned her head. Like all great champions she has retained the common touch. Only rarely will she make the slip into immodesty. "Have you ever met anyone who gained forty pounds in four days?" she asks expectantly. "That's the big time. That's major-league binging. I'm the only one I know who ever did that."

Betty, in fact, has taken that one radical step *past* the rice diet. She has had the fabled "bypass" operation, a medical procedure which ranks among the fat in approximately the same place as the famed Vincent Black Shadow holds among motorcycle freaks. It's hard to get a doctor to approve the "bypass." Kempner frowns on it severely. One must be able to convince the physician that one's obesity is an irredeemably permanent condition. Last May, after years on the rice diet, Betty was able to do this. "They figured out that if I ever got down to 120 I'd have to restrict myself to 300 calories a day just to maintain, which is totally impossible. My body works too well, it just assimilates everything I eat."

When the bypass is performed the surgeon ties off all of the lower intestine except for a foot at the top and a foot at the bottom. This leaves approximately eighteen feet of lower intestine out of work. It cuts way down the time the body has to assimilate what is ingested before it is passed on through. Since her operation Betty has dropped some 75 pounds and expects to get down to 120 in about three years.

But yes, the Turkey Caper. It was a dark and stormy night some four years ago. Betty was in the hospital on a fast. Dr. Kempner had been accusing her of cheating and she swore she wasn't, so he resolved the matter by putting her on a fast.

"I had been fasting for three and a half weeks in the hospital. I was hungrier than you can believe. It was the night before Thanksgiving. I was walking through the halls going to visit a friend in another room. When I walked past the kitchen I noticed that the door was open, which was something that *never* happened in that hospital. I looked in and lo and behold, there was row upon row of turkeys all lined up, waiting for the feast the next day. I didn't go in but continued on to my friend's room. I said to myself, 'If it's God's will that that door be open and those turkeys still be there when I come back, then it must be God's will that I have turkey for Thanksgiving.' Lo and behold they were still there. I ran to my room and put my robe on and dashed back to the kitchen. I grabbed the biggest bird I could find and stuffed it up under my nightgown. What I didn't know was that the turkeys had just been taken from the oven when I first saw them and they were still cooling. I burnt the hell out of myself but of course I couldn't tell anyone about it. How do you tell a doctor you've got turkey burns? Anyway, on the way to my room what happens but I run into a nurse. Hello, how are you feeling, she says, she wants to chat awhile. Uh, not too good, I tell her. In fact, I was just going to lie down. Feeling a little woozy, you know. What was happening, I was discovering to my horror, was that the damn turkey was leaking. I could feel this hot turkey fat dripping down my legs, and I looked down at the floor and saw this big puddle of grease forming. I got out of there quick. But before I went to my room I headed for a scale so I could weigh it. I wanted to be able to document this heist. I knew how much I weighed so I just had to subtract that from the total to find what *he* weighed. Nineteen pounds. That mother was nineteen pounds. I got back to my room at nine o'clock and started in on it. By three in the morning I had stripped his carcass clean. I was very proud. But then I had the problem of disposing of the evidence. I started flushing the bones down the toilet. Have you ever tried to flush a turkey breast down a toilet? It wouldn't fit so I finally threw it out the window. Kempner never found out. The next day when they weighed me I had gained eleven pounds. He was baffled. He never was able to figure out how someone could gain eleven pounds spontaneously. That fast was a lot of fun. Also during that time I used to send myself Candy-Grams and charge them to Kempner."

There's a stretch leading out of Durham on Roxboro Road that the ricers call Destruction Row. Some of them call it Sin Alley but the idea is the same. In the space of a couple of blocks you drive past an Arby's Roast Beef, a Kentucky Fried Chicken, Pizzaville, Dunkin' Donuts, Shoney's Big Boy, McDonald's, and Fowler's Food Store. Ground has been broken for a Sizzler Steak House. Poison. That franchise junk is bad enough for anybody, but for the rice dieters it's sheer poison. A lot of ricers will make very complicated detours just to avoid that part of town. But then there are a lot of ricers who will make very complicated detours just to get *to* Roxboro Road. Same with the Northgate Shopping Center where The Swiss Colony cheese shop offers free samples to browsers. Same with the Dairy Queen on Trinity Street and the Mayberry Ice Cream Shoppes scattered around town. Same with Gino's and Hardee's and Burger King (home of the notorious Whopper), and with the Toddle House, the Ivy Room and Howard Johnson's. Just thank God that the Baskin-Robbins is all the way over in Raleigh, although you can whiz over there for a quick hit of Jamoca Almond Fudge or English Toffee in . . . oh, no time at all.

Melody has a memory of an epic day on Destruction Row. It was New Year's Day a year ago and a bunch of ricers were sitting around this motel room, moping away with the old away-from-home holiday downs and just being hungrier than hell, which wasn't anything unusual except that somehow being hungry on a holiday adds a new dimension to it, just so god . . . damned . . . hungry they were going absolutely bonkers with food fantasies, until finally someone said, well, screw it. I mean just screw it. I'm sick of this.

I'm gonna die if I don't get something to eat. This is ridiculous. Well, that's all it took; everybody just sort of caved
in. Classic mob psychology, Melody calls it.

"I managed to resist it although I was hungry too," she
says. "Hell, you're always hungry on the rice diet, raven-
ous. I mean it's really a bitch. But I was just dead set against
cheating. I was losing really good at the time and I was so
damned tired of being fat that I wasn't going to cheat for
anything. But I was the only one who had a car and they
wanted to binge. I didn't mind driving them around even
though I knew I was going to be sorely tempted."

So they all jumped into Melody's car and headed out to
Destruction Row. Okay, where do you want to hit first?
Melody asks them. Listen, says this chick Margo in the back
seat who was, Melody says, really a blimp, it doesn't matter
where we hit first because before this is over we're gonna
hit 'em all anyway. Just pull in somewhere, Melody, for
Christ's sake.

"Oh man, you wouldn't *believe* it. I mean I've been a
gorger all my life but I'd never seen anything like this. You
figure here's five people, *really* fat, their whole lives have
been centered around food. And here they've been on this
really brutal starvation diet for months, maybe doing a little
minor cheating here and there but no big thing, you know?
And all of a sudden they collectively decide to pull out all
the stops. Maybe they wouldn't have gone off the deep end
like this by themselves, I don't know, but wow, they were
all in it together, you know, like a band of thieves or school
kids on a tear or something. That car was carrying a lot of
accumulated hunger. We went from Pizzaville to Colonel
Sanders over to McDonald's then back to Dunkin' Donuts,
just getting bags and bags of this junk. *Rabid.* And as far
as I could see they were totally guiltless. It had come to
that. We drove around for a couple of hours while they
consumed all this stuff, which by the way was driving me
mad, but I held out, God knows how. Then somebody said
that since we had gone this far we should head over to

Howard Johnson's for some sundaes. You know, let's do it up right. That's when the first pangs of guilt started to set in. Like two of the girls decided to *split* a hot fudge sundae instead of having one apiece. A little atonement, you know. Of course they each had a couple of brownies to help get it down."

From THE LIFE AND TIMES OF WILLIAM HOWARD TAFT

by Henry F. Pringle

Although he was a witty and distinguished president, William Howard Taft earned at least one distinction which did not please him. He was this country's fattest president.

In *The Life and Times of William Howard Taft* (New York: Farrar & Rinehart, Inc., 1939), official biographer Henry F. Pringle offers details of Taft's struggle with his own bulk.

On page 155, he writes: "Taft did not go to [the Spanish-American] war because he was the antithesis of the Rooseveltian doctrine of strenuosity. He was growing more and more stout by the year. Exertion, to Taft, had but one purpose; the reduction of flesh."

Taft writes home, on a visit made to Japan in 1900, and described by Pringle:

> During the long days at sea . . . Taft, worried about his bulk, exercised by tramping around the deck. His weight both amused and annoyed him when he rode, for the first time, in the jinrickishas on shore. The party had visited the temples at Nikko, high in the mountains:
>
> "The road was steep and got steeper. I had one 'pusher' in addition to the jinrickisha man when I began, another joined when we were halfway up, and it seemed to me that [when] we struck the last hill the whole village was engaged in the push. The Japanese seemed to look upon me with great amusement; at the various places where we changed cars there were a great number of people clattering along on their wooden platforms which they use as shoes, and they gathered in crowds about me, smiling and enjoying the prospect of so much flesh and size."

Pringle offers a complete record of one of Taft's attempts to diet. The great man is determined to lose flesh and does so but the record leaves some room for speculation as the month of January is, mysteriously, missing. We must assume that Taft behaved himself from Christmas until February 3, because he managed to drop almost twenty pounds in that period, but the imagination lingers at laden Christmas tables, holiday eggnog parties and lavish New Year's Eve festivities. Pringle writes:

> Taft's new efficiency included zealous attention to physical fitness. "I will make a conscientious effort to lose flesh," he promised. "I am convinced that this undue drowsiness is due to the accumulation of flesh . . . were I appointed to the bench I fear I could not keep awake in my present condition." He rode horseback almost daily. In December, 1905, he began a diet under the supervision of Dr. N. E. Yorke-Davis of London, and the results were as astonishing as they were beneficial. On the S.S. *Korea,* returning from his visit to the Philippines that year, he had weighed 326 pounds. The secretary of war submitted daily reports on his vanishing weight. It was a gallant record:

1905			
Dec. 1st		Dressed 7 P.M.	320-3/4
1905		Stripped	
Dec.	2	7 A.M.	314-3/4
"	3	9:30 A.M.	313
"	4	8:30 A.M.	312-1/2
"	5	8:30 A.M.	312-1/8
"	6	8:30 A.M.	311
"	7	8:30 A.M.	312-3/4
"	9	8:30 A.M.	312
"	9	8:30 A.M.	310
"	10	Absent from home	
"	11	8:30 A.M.	309-1/8
"	12	"	308-1/2
"	13	"	308-1/4
"	14	"	307-3/4
"	15	"	305-7/8
"	16	"	305-15/16
"	17	"	304-3/4
"	18	"	303-15/16
1906			
Feb.	3	8:45	284
"	4	9:30	283-9/16
"	5	9:00	282-7/8

" 6	8:45	282-9/16
" 7	8:45	282-1/16
" 8	8:45	282-1/16
" 9	8:15	281-7/8
" 10	8:30	281-7/8
" 11	In New York	
" 12	Before 9:00	281-3/4
" 13	" "	281-5/8
" 14	" "	281-3/4
" 15	" "	280-3/4
" 16	" "	282
" 17	" "	281
" 18	9 A.M.	279-1/2
Mar. 12	9:15	267-1/4
" 13	9:15	266-11/16
" 14	In New York	
Mar. 15	In New York	
" 16	9:00	266-5/8
" 17	9:15	266-15/16
" 18	9:30	266-5/16
" 19	9:00	267-1/2
" 20	9:00	266-5/8
" 21	9:10	265-13/16
" 22	9:00	264-15/16
" 23	8:45	265-3/4

By the middle of April, 1906, he was down to 255¾ pounds. That summer he weighed only 250 pounds, by no means too much for a man Taft's height and build. His health, of course, was infinitely improved. His digestion was better. At no time, despite the rather drastic reduction, had he experienced the slightest discomfort. But his pocketbook felt it. "I have had to pay . . . $400 for clothes alterations, etc., so you see that considering my bills for medical advice and my tailor's bill, a reduction of seventy pounds is not an inexpensive luxury," he told Mrs. Taft.

Pringle continues, describing the variation in Taft's weight and relating it to stresses in his life:

The Chief Justice had reason to be concerned about his health. Like all men whose weight is excessive, he lacked a normal resistance to organic diseases and his heart, pumping blood through his mountainous body, had been gravely strained for many years. Taft was a temperate man in all ways but one. He did not use alcohol. He did not smoke. He did not stay up late and sacrifice sleep. His only dissipation was food and surely, in so big a man, this was a human fault. At times he conquered even that. Returning to the United States early in 1904 to become secretary of war, he had weighed 326 pounds. By dieting and exercise, he had cut this to 250 pounds in somewhat over two years. He fell from virtue in the White House, though; he had too many other problems to bother with weight. Indeed, it is almost possible to plot relating curves on Taft's weight and happiness. When he was contented, his weight went down because he paid attention to it. When he was bothered, his bulk increased. Thus he dieted after leaving the presidency and its worries in 1913. He was careful again when he was chief justice. He congratulated himself, a year before he died, that he weighed just 244 pounds. On graduating from Yale in 1878, he noted, the figure had been 243 and his doctors thought that 240 to 250 pounds was about right.

Writing to a friend in 1924, Taft reflects on his failing health: "I think I have been just what I have been—a damn fool in many ways. . . . I have thought . . . that my strength was equal to anything, and I found that it was not."

BOULE DE SUIF

by *Guy de Maupassant*

Translated by *Carl A. Viggiani*

Day after day bits and pieces of the shattered army made their way through the town. They were disorganized hordes of men, not disciplined soldiers. They had long dirty beards; their uniforms were rags, and they moved ahead listlessly, no flags and no officers leading them. They were crushed, exhausted, unable to think or act, walking as if by force of habit and falling over with fatigue every time they stopped. Most were reservists, peace-loving people with small incomes, bending under the weight of their rifles; there were alert little militiamen, as subject to fear as to patriotic enthusiasm, as quick to attack the enemy as to run; then, following them, a few infantrymen in red breeches, the remains of a division chewed up in a fierce battle; artillery-men in dark coats walking alongside the foot-soldiers; and here and there one could see the shining helmets of booted cavalrymen who were having trouble keeping up with the brisker pace of the line soldiers.

Units of partisans with heroic names—"Vengeurs de la Défaite"—"Citoyens de la Tombe"—"Partageurs de la Mort"—passed by in turn, looking like bandits.

Their officers, grain merchants, drapers, chandlers and soap merchants, all soldiers of circumstance appointed to their ranks because of their money or their long moustaches, weighed down by their weapons and their fine flannel uniforms and gold braid, boasted loudly, discussed battle plans and led one to believe they were the only hope of dying France; but they were sometimes afraid of their own troops who, while often brave above and beyond the call of duty, were nevertheless thieving and lecherous gal-lows-birds.

It was rumored that the Prussians were about to enter Rouen.

National Guardsmen, who for two months had scouted the surrounding woods with the utmost prudence—occasionally shooting their own sentries—and who would rush for their weapons at the sound of a rabbit in the brush, had gone home. Their guns, their uniforms, all the deadly equipment that had only recently spread terror along the highways for eight miles around, had suddenly vanished from the scene.

The last French troops had just crossed the Seine on their way to Pont-Audemer through Saint-Sever and Bourg-Achard; following them, on foot between his two orderlies, came their despairing commanding general, un-able to organize any resistance with these motley remnants, bewildered like everyone else by the collapse of a nation used to winning but now disastrously beaten in spite of its legendary courage.

Then a deep calm, a silent dread settled over the city. Pot-bellied bourgeois, castrated by their years in business, anxiously awaited their conquerors, quaking with fear lest their roasting spits and kitchen knives be considered to be weapons by the enemy.

Life had come to a stop; shops were closed, the streets were deserted. Occasionally a Rouennais, frightened by the silence, could be seen speeding by, hugging the walls.

The anguish of waiting makes people yearn for the en-emy.

The afternoon of the day following the departure of the French troops, a few Uhlans, who seemed to materialize from thin air, streaked through the town. A little later, a dark mass of troops descended St. Catherine's Hill as two columns of invaders appeared along the roads from Dar-netal and Boisguillaume. At precisely the same moment the advance guards of three army corps converged on the Square of the Hôtel de Ville and from all the adjoining streets came the German army, its endless battalions making the pavement ring with their metallic rhythmic step.

Orders shouted in foreign guttural voices rose along the dead and deserted houses, while behind the shuttered windows eyes peered out at the victors, now masters of the city and of their lives and wealth by "right of war." In their darkened bedrooms, the inhabitants of Rouen were suffering the terror provoked by cataclysms like murderous earthquakes, against which all wisdom and strength are powerless. The same feeling arises each time the established order of things is upset, when security disappears, or when everything protected by the laws of men and nature falls to the mercy of irrational and ferocious brutality. Earthquakes that bury whole populations under their cities; ravaging floods that carry away drowned peasants, the corpses of oxen and roof-beams in one violent movement; or the proud armies that massacre those who resist and take all the others prisoner, pillaging in the name of the Sword and thanking God to the sound of cannon; such are the terrifying plagues that destroy all belief in Eternal Justice and all the trust we are taught in the protection of Heaven and Human Reason.

Soon, however, small detachments of soldiers were seen knocking at doors and disappearing into houses. First the invasion, and now the occupation. The conquered were now obliged to be gracious to their conquerors. Once their initial terror had subsided, a new calm set in. In many homes Prussian officers ate with the family. Some were well-bred, politely expressed sympathy for France, and said how repugnant they found this war. People expressed gratitude for this delicate sentiment; besides, one never knew when their protection might be needed. By handling them diplomatically they might even be able to cut down the number of men quartered in the town. Besides, why insult someone when you are totally at his mercy? That wouldn't be bravery; it would be recklessness. And recklessness was no longer a weakness of the bourgeois of Rouen, as it was during the heroic defense that made the city illustrious. And lastly (this was the crowning argument, inspired by French urbanity), it was after all still proper to be polite to the enemy in your home provided you weren't friendly with him in public. On the streets they ignored one another, but indoors they chatted amiably, and the Germans stayed later every evening to warm themselves at the family hearth.

Little by little the town itself began to look normal again. The French still didn't go out very much, but the streets swarmed with Prussian soldiers. The Blue Hussard officers who dragged their long sabers along the pavement didn't seem to be any more contemptuous of the citizenry than the French light cavalry officers who had drunk in the same cafés the year before.

But there was something subtle and unfamiliar abroad, a strange and unbearable atmosphere, like a penetrating odor—the odor of invasion. It filled every home and public place, changed the taste of food, and made people feel as if they were in a distant foreign land among dangerous and barbaric tribes.

The conquerors demanded money, a lot of money. The inhabitants of Rouen paid; besides, they were rich. But the more affluent a Norman becomes the more he suffers from any sacrifice at all, from the loss of any bit of the fortune he sees passing into someone else's hands.

But seven or eight miles downstream, toward Croisset, Dieppedalle and Biessart, bargemen and fishermen often dredged up the corpse of a bloated German, knifed or beaten to death, his skull crushed, or kicked into the stream from a bridge. The mud of the river-bed buried these clandestine and savage but legitimate acts of vengeance, these silent attacks, far more dangerous than battles in broad daylight and without the promise of glory.

Hatred of the foreign enemy will always inspire a few heroes to die for an idea.

But in the end, since the invaders, even while subjecting the town to their harsh discipline, didn't commit any of the atrocities that had been attributed to them all along their triumphal march, people took courage and merchants once again turned their hearts and minds to business. A few had important investments in Le Havre and decided to try to reach the port city by going overland to Dieppe and taking a boat from there.

They used their influence with German officers they knew and soon obtained a permit to leave from the commanding general.

They engaged a four-horse coach (ten persons reserved places with the carrier) and decided to leave on a Tuesday morning before dawn in order to avoid being seen.

For some time now the ground had been hardened by frost, and on Monday, toward three o'clock, large black clouds from the north brought snow that fell all that evening and through the night.

At four-thirty in the morning the travellers met in the courtyard of the Hôtel de Normandie, where they were to take the coach.

They were still half asleep and stood shivering in their wraps. In the darkness it was hard to recognize anyone: the layers of heavy winter clothing made them all look like fat priests in long cassocks. But two men did recognize each other, a third came up to them, and they began to chat: "I'm taking my wife," said one. "So am I." "I too." The first man added: "We're not coming back to Rouen. And if the Prussians reach Le Havre we'll go to England." Being very much alike, they all had the same plans.

Meantime, the horses hadn't been harnessed. From time to time a groom carrying a lantern would appear in one doorway and disappear into another. Horses' hooves struck the ground, the sound deadened by the stable-litter, the voice of a man talking to the animals and cursing could be heard coming from the stable. A gentle murmur of bells signalled that the horses were being harnessed; the murmur became a clear and continuous rustle, punctuated by the horses' movements, stopped from time to time, then rose again in a burst, accompanied by the dead sound of a horse's hoof striking the ground.

The door suddenly closed. Then silence. The freezing bourgeois said nothing; they stood by, waiting, stiff and motionless.

A solid curtain of snowflakes sparkled endlessly as it fell; it wiped out all forms and shapes and powdered everything with a frozen foam; in the deep silence of the sleeping town buried under winter, the only sound that could be heard was the vague, ineffable and floating rustle of falling snow, more a sensation than a sound, an intermingling of weight-less atoms that seemed to fill all space and blanket the world.

The man reappeared, carrying his lantern and leading a melancholy and reluctant horse. He moved the horse up to the pole, fastened the traces, took quite a while to secure the harness because he had only one hand free. As he was about to get the second horse, he noticed all the motionless travellers, by now whitened by the snow, and said: "Get in the coach; you'll at least be under cover."

It hadn't occurred to them, probably, but now they rushed in. The three men settled their wives into the far end of the coach, then got in; other indistinct and veiled shapes took the last seats in their turn without exchanging a word.

Their feet sank into the thick layer of straw covering the coach floor. The ladies at the far end had brought little copper foot-warmers filled with charcoal; they lit them and for a while they detailed the virtues of foot-warmers in subdued tones, telling each other things they all had known from some time.

Finally, the coach was ready. Because of the snow, six horses instead of four had been harnessed. A voice from outside asked: "Everyone here?" A voice from the interior answered: "Yes." They left.

The vehicle moved slowly. The wheels sank into the snow and the whole chassis creaked and groaned complain-ingly; the horses slipped, blew, and smoked and the coach-man's gigantic whip cracked continually, flying to all sides. Coiling and uncoiling like a long thin snake, it would suddenly slice into one or another of six round croups which would stiffen with a violent effort to move forward.

Night turned imperceptibly into day. Those light snow-flakes, which one traveller—a pure-breed Rouennais—compared to a rain of cotton, had stopped falling. A gray light filtered through big, dark, heavy clouds that heightened the brilliant whiteness of the countryside, in which one could see now a stand of tall frost-covered trees, now a cottage hooded with snow.

In the coach, the travellers looked at each other with curiosity in the sad light of dawn.

At the far end of the coach, in the best seats, Monsieur and Madame Loiseau, wholesale wine-merchants of the Rue Grand-Pont, dozed opposite each other.

Once a salesman for a merchant who went bankrupt, Loiseau bought the man's business and made a fortune. He sold abominable wine at very low prices to small country retailers and was known among his friends and acquaintances as a sly rogue, a real Norman, full of cunning and joviality.

His reputation as a swindler was so well established that one evening at the Prefecture, Monsieur Tournel, author of fables and songs, possessed of a sharp and biting wit, in short the pride of Rouen, seeing the ladies about to fall asleep, proposed a game of "Loiseau vole."* His pun flew through the Prefect's reception rooms and then through town, and for a month provincial wags howled with laughter at Loiseau.

Loiseau was also famous for practical jokes of all kinds, good and bad, and no one could mention his name without immediately adding: "Oh, that Loiseau, he's priceless."

He was rather small, had a balloon-shaped belly topped by a ruddy face, and sported graying mutton-chops.

His wife was tall, stout, resolute, loud and decisive and

---

*Pun on the words *l'oiseau,* "the bird," and *vole,* "flies," "steals."

she contributed order and accurate accounting to his business, which he enlivened with his joyful playfulness.

Beside them sat (with somewhat greater dignity, since he belonged to a higher caste) Monsieur Carré-Lamadon, a man of some importance: a cotton magnate, owner of three spinning-mills, Officer of the Legion of Honor and member of the General Council. Under Napoleon he had remained a member of the loyal opposition simply in order to exact a greater price for rallying to the cause that he fought, to use his expression, with "blunted arms." Madame Carré-Lamadon, much younger than her husband, was the consolation of the officers of good family assigned to the Rouen garrison.

Dainty, pretty, huddled in her furs, she sat facing her husband and gazed mournfully at the pitiful interior of the coach.

Her neighbors, Count and Countess Hubert de Bréville, bore one of the oldest and noblest names in Normandy. The Count, an elderly and aristocratic gentleman, did his best to emphasize by every artifice of dress his natural resemblance to King Henry IV; according to a legend in which the family took great pride, Henry IV had fathered the illegitimate child of a lady de Bréville and her husband had in consequences become a Count and provincial governor.

Count Hubert, a colleague of Monsieur Carré-Lamadon in the General Council, represented the Orleanist party in the Department. His marriage to the daughter of a small ship-owner from Nantes had always been a mystery. But since the Countess had a noble bearing, entertained better than any, and even was rumored to have been the mistress of one of King Louis-Philippe's sons, the provincial nobility honored her and her salon was the most important one in the region—the only one that preserved the ancient traditions of gallantry and to which entrée was difficult.

It was said that the Bréville fortune, all in property, amounted to about five hundred thousand pounds.

These six people occupied the far side of the coach, the side representing wealthy gentility, serene in its power and blessed with Religion and Principles.

By some strange chance all the ladies were on one side; the Countess sat next to two nuns who spent the time telling their beads and mumbling Paternosters and Aves. One was rather old and her face was so disfigured by small-pox that she looked as if she had received a charge of grape-shot point-blank. The other, quite frail, had a pretty and sickly face and the chest of a consumptive burning with the kind of faith that makes martyrs and mystics.

Sitting opposite them were a man and a woman who attracted everyone's attention.

The man was very well known: he was Cornudet "the Demo," the terror of respectable people. For twenty years he had soaked his great red beard in the beer-mugs of every republican café in the region. With his comrades he had squandered a rather large fortune inherited from his father—a confectioner—and now he impatiently awaited the coming of the Republic and the position he had earned in so many revolutionary drinking bouts. On September 4, perhaps as a result of a practical joke, he was led to understand that he had been named Prefect; when he tried to assume his post, however, the clerks who had taken over the Prefecture refused to acknowledge his authority and he was forced to withdraw. He was a good chap, harmless and obliging, and he had worked with incomparable zeal in organizing the defense of Rouen. He'd had trenches dug in the flat country, had all the young adjoining forest trees cut down as road-blocks, he'd strewn traps on all the highways, and as the enemy approached, completely satisfied with his preparations, had quickly withdrawn to the town. He now thought he could make himself more useful in Le Havre, where fresh defenses would soon be needed.

The woman, one of the so-called "ladies of the night," was famous for a precocious rotundity that had earned her the nickname Boule de Suif, "Ball of Fat." She was petite, round, and soft as goose-fat, her fingers were pudgy and squeezed in at the joints, like strings of little pork sausages; her skin was taut and shiny and she had enormous breasts that threatened to burst through her dress, but she was very appetizing and much sought-after because her youthful freshness gave men such pleasure. Her face was a little round apple, a peony bud about to bloom; she had magnificent glowing black eyes protected by long thick lashes which made them look shadowy; and below them, sweet, small, wet and inviting lips that opened to reveal tiny milk-white teeth.

She possessed, in addition, many inestimable qualities, it was said. As soon as they recognized her, the respectable women began to whisper, but the words "prostitute" and "public shame" were whispered so loudly that she looked up. She then swept her neighbors with such a provocative and bold look that they fell silent and lowered their eyes, all but Loiseau, who watched her with a twinkle in his eye.

Soon the conversation picked up again between the three ladies, whom this girl's presence had suddenly turned into friends, almost intimates. They seemed to feel it their matronly duty to build a wall against this tart, for legalized love always looks with scorn on its licentious sister.

The three men were also brought closer together, but by a conservative instinct aroused by the sight of Cornudet, and they talked money with a certain tone of contempt for the poor. Count Hubert talked about the damage done to his properties by the Prussians, and the losses that would result from stolen cattle and lost harvests, with the self-assurance of a great lord who was ten times a millionaire and whom this devastation might inconvenience for perhaps a year. Monsieur Carré-Lamadon, whose cotton interests had sustained severe losses, had prudently sent six hundred thousand francs to England for the rainy day he always expected to come. As for Loiseau, he had managed to sell all of the mediocre wine that remained in his cellars to the French Quartermaster Corps, so the Government owed him a huge sum of money that he expected to be paid in Le Havre.

All three exchanged rapid and friendly looks. Although they belonged to different castes, they felt themselves brothers in money, members of that great freemasonry of the rich whose pockets jingle with the sound of gold whenever they put their hands in them.

The coach went so slowly that by ten in the morning they hadn't gone eight miles. The men had gotten out three times and climbed the hills on foot. They began to worry because they were supposed to lunch at Tôtes and they now had no hope of getting there even by nightfall. Everyone was watching for a roadside inn when suddenly the coach got stuck in a snowbank and it took two hours to get it out.

Their appetite increased and made them edgy; not an inn or tavern could be found open, because the approach of the Prussians and the passage of starved French troops had frightened away all tradespeople.

The gentlemen looked for food in farmhouses along the road, but they didn't even find bread: suspicious peasants were hiding their reserves for fear of being pillaged by starving soldiers who simply took any food they found.

Around one, Loiseau complained that he had a painful hollow in his stomach. Everyone else had been suffering just like him for some time; and the increasingly sharp hunger pangs killed all conversation.

From time to time someone yawned; someone else would imitate him; and all, each according to his character, *savoir-vivre* and social position would open his mouth either noisily or discreetly, quickly putting his hand in front of the gaping hole from which a cloud of vapor issued.

Boule de Suif bent over several times as if she were looking for something under her skirt. She would hesitate a second, look at her neighbors, then sit up again quietly. Everyone around her looked pale and drawn. Loiseau declared that he would pay a thousand francs for a ham. His wife made a gesture as if to protest the expenditure but quickly sat still again. She always suffered when she heard talk of money being wasted and couldn't even understand jokes on the subject. "The fact is that I don't feel well," the Count said. "Why didn't I think of bringing food along?" They all blamed themselves in the same way.

But Cornudet had a flask of rum; he offered it around and was coldly refused by all. Except Loiseau, who took a sip and said, as he returned the flask: "That's really good; it warms you up and makes you forget you're hungry." The alcohol put him into a gay mood and he suggested they do what they did on the little boat in the song—namely eat the fattest passenger. This sly reference to Boule de Suif shocked the ladies and gentlemen. They didn't answer; but Cornudet smiled. The two nuns had stopped mumbling their rosary and sat stock-still, their hands stuck into their wide sleeves, their eyes obstinately lowered, probably offering back to heaven the sacrifice of pain it had sent them.

Finally, around three o'clock, as they were crossing an interminable plain, without a single village in sight, Boule de Suif bent over quickly and took from under the seat a large basket covered with a white napkin.

First she took out a little faience plate and a fine silver drinking cup, then a huge terrine containing two chickens *en gelée*; inside the basket one could also see other carefully wrapped delicacies, pâtés, fruit, sweets, enough food for a three-day trip so that tavern cuisine could be avoided. The necks of four bottles stuck out between the little packets of food. She took a chicken breast and began to eat it, delicately, with a roll called a "Régence" in Normandy.

Everyone turned toward her. Then the odor of the food spread, nostrils dilated, mouths watered abundantly and jaws were painfully clenched. The contempt the ladies felt for this girl became ferocious; they wanted to kill her, throw her out of the coach, leave her in the snow with her drinking cup, her basket and her food.

But Loiseau was eating up the terrine with his eyes. He said, "Splendid, Madame. You have been more prudent than we. There are people who think of everything." She turned toward him: "Would you care to have some, Sir?

It's hard to go without eating all day." He bowed: "Upon my word, I won't say no. I can't stand it any longer. Besides, we've got to rough it, don't we, Madame?" And, looking around at his fellow passengers, he added: "At times like this it's good to find generous people." He spread a newspaper on his lap and with a pocket knife he always carried with him speared a chicken leg entirely covered with glaze, bit off a piece and chewed it with such gusto that a chorus of deep sighs of distress filled the coach.

Boule de Suif humbly and sweetly invited the nuns to share her meal. They both accepted on the spot and without even looking up began to eat after a few mumbled thanks. Cornudet also accepted his neighbor's offer and the four of them made a table on their knees with some newspapers.

Mouths opened and bit into the food and, without stopping, swallowed, chewed, gulped with a kind of ferocity. Off in the corner, Loiseau was also hard at work and whispering to his wife to follow his example. She resisted for a long time, but after a long sharp hunger pain she gave in. Her husband then asked his "charming companion" in polite and elegant terms if she would allow him to offer a piece of chicken to his wife. With a friendly smile she said, "Of course, my good Sir," and held the terrine out to him.

There was a moment of embarrassment when the first bottle of Bordeaux was opened: there was only one cup. They passed it around, wiping it clean after they drank. Only Cornudet, probably out of a flirtatious gallantry, placed his lips where Boule de Suif had drunk.

Then, surrounded by people who were eating, and sick from the odor of food, Count and Countess de Bréville as well as Monsieur and Madame Carré-Lamadon suffered that odious torture that still bears the name of Tantalus. Suddenly the manufacturer's young wife sighed so loudly that everyone looked at her; she was as white as the snow; her eyes closed, her head dropped. She had fainted. In a panic, her husband begged his companions to help. They all lost their heads except the older nun, who held her up, forced Boule de Suif's cup between her lips and made her swallow a few drops of wine. The pretty lady stirred, opened her eyes, smiled and declared feebly that she felt very well now. But the nun made her drink a whole glass of Bordeaux so it wouldn't happen again, adding: "You're just hungry; that's all that's wrong with you."

Then Boule de Suif, blushing with embarrassment, looked at the other four passengers and stammered: "Dear me, I don't know if I dare offer you ladies and gentlemen . . ." She fell silent, afraid that she might insult them. But Loiseau spoke up: "Why of course! In moments like these we are all brothers and sisters and we must help each other. Come, ladies, don't stand on ceremony, accept, for goodness' sake! We don't know if we'll find an inn even by nightfall. At this rate we won't get to Tôtes before tomorrow noon." They hesitated; no one dared assume the responsibility of saying yes.

But the Count settled the matter. He turned to the intimidated little fat girl, and, assuming his most aristocratic air, he said: "Madame, we accept with gratitude."

The first step was the hardest. Once they had crossed their Rubicon they went at the food with a vengeance. They emptied the contents of the basket: a pâté de foie gras, a lark pâté, a piece of smoked tongue, Crassane pears, a square of Pont-l'Evêque, petits-fours, and a jar of pickled gherkins and onions (Boule de Suif, like all women, loved appetizers).

They didn't feel they could eat this girl's food without talking to her, however. So they chatted with her, a little stiffly at first, but then more freely as they realized she knew her place. Madame de Bréville and Madame Carré-Lamadon, both tactful ladies, were delicate and gracious with her. The Countess especially was able to communicate that friendly condescension of noble ladies who can't be soiled by any contact, and she was absolutely charming. But stout Madame Loiseau, who had the soul of a gendarme, remained ill-tempered, said practically nothing but ate a lot.

Naturally, they talked about the war. They told stories about Prussian atrocities and heroic exploits of the French; all these people who were running away from the enemy paid homage to the courage of others. They soon began to talk about personal experiences and Boule de Suif told with deep emotion, and with the eloquence that girls sometimes have when they get carried away, why she had left Rouen: "At first I thought I could stay. I had plenty of food in the house and I thought it would be better to feed a few soldiers than to leave town and end up God knows where. But when I saw those Prussians I couldn't do it. My blood boiled and I cried with shame all day. Believe me, if I were a man. . . . I watched those fat pigs in their pointed helmets from my window and my maid had to hold me to keep me from throwing my furniture on them as they marched by. Then some were billeted in my house, but when they arrived I jumped at the throat of the first one through the door. They're no harder to strangle than anyone else! And I would've finished him off if they hadn't dragged me away by the hair. I had to hide after that. Finally, when I had a chance, I left, and here I am."

They all congratulated her. She was growing in the esteem of her companions, none of whom had been as plucky as she. Cornudet smiled approvingly as he listened, like a benign apostle; it was the smile of a priest hearing the praise of God from the lips of a true believer, for all long-bearded partisans of democracy have a monopoly on patriotism, as priests have a monopoly on religion. When his turn came he spoke dogmatically and with the bombast learned from government proclamations pasted on the walls every day, and he climaxed his tirade with a bravura piece of elegance in which he gave a masterful verbal drubbing to "that scum Badinguet."

But that made Boule de Suif furious because she was a Bonapartist. Her face turned beet-red and she stammered indignantly, "I'd like to have seen you and your kind in his place. *That* would have been a filthy mess. It was you who betrayed *him*, poor man. If we were ever governed by ras-

cals like you there would be only one thing left to do—leave
France." Cornudet, seemingly unmoved, gave her a contemptuous and superior smile, and as the company sensed
insults and foul language about to explode, the Count came
between them and calmed the exasperated young girl, not
without difficulty, and proclaimed that all sincere political
opinions should be respected. But the Countess and the
manufacturer's wife, who harbored the irrational hatred of
nice people for the Republic and nourished that instinctive
affection all women have for despotic military leaders like
Napoleon, were drawn in spite of themselves to this prostitute of such great dignity, whose political beliefs bore such
a strong resemblance to theirs.

The basket was empty. The ten of them had finished off
its contents without any trouble at all, and now they regretted that it wasn't bigger. The conversation continued for
a while, but became lukewarm as the food disappeared.

Night fell, they were soon in complete darkness, and the
cold—always sharper during digestion—made Boule de
Suif shiver, despite her thick layer of fat. Madame de
Bréville kindly offered her her foot-warmer, which had
been filled with charcoal several times since morning; the
offer was accepted immediately, for Boule de Suif's feet
were freezing. Madame Carré-Lamadon and Madame Loiseau gave theirs to the nuns.

The coachman had lit his lanterns. They cast a bright
light on a cloud of vapor that rose from the sweating croups
of the wheel-horses and on the blanket of snow that seemed
to unroll on both sides of the road under the moving reflection of the lights.

Inside the coach nothing could be seen; but there was
a sudden quick movement where Boule de Suif and Cornudet sat, and Loiseau, whose eyes searched the darkness,
thought he saw the long-bearded man move quickly to the
side as if he had gotten a good but silent kick in the shins.

Tiny lights were now visible ahead. It was Tôtes. They
had been on the road for eleven hours, which with the two
hours to feed and rest the horses made thirteen in all. The

coach entered the town and stopped in front of the Hôtel du Commerce.

The coach door was opened, finally! A familiar sound made the passengers shudder: it was the ring of a scabbard against the ground. At the same moment, the voice of a German shouted something.

Although the coach had stopped, no one got out, as if they expected to be massacred as they stepped down. Then the coachman appeared, holding in his hand one of the coach lanterns, which suddenly lit up the whole interior of the vehicle with its two rows of terrified faces, open mouths and eyes staring with surprise and fright.

A German officer, brightly illuminated, stood next to the coachman; he was a tall young man, extremely slender, blond, squeezed into his uniform like a girl in her corset, and, with his flat shiny cap on the side of his head, he looked like a bell-boy in an English hotel. His moustache of long straight hairs, thinning gradually on either side into single blond hairs that were so fine as to be imperceptible, seemed to weigh down the corners of his mouth and to pull down his cheeks as well, making his lips appear to sag.

In an Alsatian French accent he invited the travellers to come out, saying stiffly: "Please be kind enough to step down."

The nuns were the first to obey, with the docility of saintly women accustomed to submissiveness. The Count and Countess came next, followed by the manufacturer and his wife; then Loiseau, pushing his larger half before him. As he stepped down Loiseau said, "God day, Sir," more out of prudence than politeness. The latter, insolent like all men who feel omnipotent, looked at him without even answering.

Although Boule de Suif and Cornudet were nearest the door, they came out last, but with an air of solemnity and pride before the enemy. The fat girl tried to control herself and stay calm: the "Demo" stroked his long reddish beard gravely, but with a slight quiver in his hand. They wanted above all to maintain their dignity, being fully aware that in these encounters they represented their fatherland. They were both disgusted by their companions' servility: Boule de Suif tried to maintain an attitude of proud dignity that set her off from the ladies of quality, while Cornudet, feeling he had to set an example, by his attitude continued the mission of resistance that he had begun by blocking the roads to Rouen.

They entered the inn and went into the vast kitchen where the German, having looked at the travel pass signed by the commanding general, on which were stated the name, description and profession of each passenger, scrutinized each member of the party, comparing them with their written descriptions.

Then he said brusquely: "Very well," and withdrew.

They breathed a sigh of relief. Since they were still hungry they ordered supper. It would be a half hour before they could be served, so while the servants busied themselves with the meal the travellers went to have a look at their rooms. They were all located on one long corridor that ended with a glass door with a large number on it.

Finally, they were about to sit down to supper when the innkeeper himself appeared. He was a former horse-dealer, a big man suffering from asthma, hoarse, always wheezing and clearing his throat. His father had blessed him with the name Follenvie.

He asked: "Is Mademoiselle Elisabeth Rousset here?"

Boule de Suif gave a start: "I'm Mademoiselle Rousset."

"Mademoiselle, the Prussian officer wants to speak to you immediately."

"To me?"

"Yes, if you are Mademoiselle Elisabeth Rousset."

She was confused for a moment, but quickly recovered and said: "That may be, but I won't go."

There was a stir around her: everyone had an opinion, everyone wondered what the order was all about. The Count came up to her:

"Madame, you're making a mistake. If you refuse you can cause a lot of trouble not only for yourself but also for your companions. It doesn't pay to resist people who are stronger than you. There would be no danger in obeying; it's probably some formality that he forgot."

Everybody agreed and they begged her, urged her, lectured her and finally persuaded her to go; they were all afraid of the unpleasant consequences her stubbornness could produce. She said finally:

"I'll do it, but only because you insist."

The Countess took her hand:

"And we thank you."

She left. They waited for her to come back before sitting down to table.

They were all upset that they weren't called instead of this irascible and passionate girl and mentally prepared a string of platitudes just in case they were to be called too.

After about ten minutes she came back, out of breath, red with rage, exasperated. She blurted: "The scum, the filthy scum!"

They were eager to know what had happened, but she refused to speak; as the Count persisted in asking, she answered with great dignity: "No, it has nothing to do with you, but I can't tell you what it's about."

So they sat down around a great soup tureen fragrant with the odor of cabbage. Despite this brief moment of alarm they supped gaily. The cider was good, so the nuns and Monsieur and Madame Loiseau ordered some, for reasons of economy. The others ordered wine, Cornudet beer. He had a particular way of opening the beer-bottle, making the beer bubble up, examining it by tipping the glass, which he then raised against the light to appraise its color. When he drank, his great beard, whose color resembled the color of his favorite drink, quivered with tenderness; he squinted in order to keep sight of his tankard and he seemed to be fulfilling the only function for which he was born. You would have said that he had established both an analogy and an affinity in his mind between the two great passions that filled his life: Pale Ale and the Revolution; and it was clear that he couldn't drink one without thinking of the other.

Monsieur and Madame Follenvie sat at the other end of the table. Wheezing like a dying locomotive, Follenvie was too short of breath to talk as he ate, but his wife never stopped. She described all her experiences with the Prussians, what they did, what they said; she hated them, first, because they cost her money and, second, because she had two sons in the army. She addressed herself mainly to the Countess because she felt flattered to talk to a lady of quality.

Then she lowered her voice to talk about more delicate matters, and her husband interrupted her now and then: "You'd do better to be still, Madame Follenvie." But she paid no attention and went right on:

"Yes, Madame, all they eat is pig and potatoes, and sometimes potatoes and pig. And don't you think they're clean. Oh, no. They make a mess everywhere they go, if you'll forgive my saying so. And you should see them drill, hour after hour, day after day. There they are, in some field; forward march, to the rear march, column right and column left. . . . If only they tilled the land, or worked on the roads back home. But no, soldiers are of no value to anyone. Why should poor people feed them while they learn how to kill? . . . I'm only a poor ignorant woman, it's true, but when I see them wearing themselves out marching up and down from morning to evening, I say to myself: When there are people who spend their lives making discoveries that will help others, why must there be so many who go to so much trouble to hurt their fellow-men? Really, isn't it an abomination to kill people, whether they're Prussians or Englishmen or Poles, or Frenchman? . . . If you take revenge against someone who has done you harm, that's bad, because you're condemned for it, but when they kill our children with guns, as if they were game, that's good, since they decorate the ones who kill the most? No, you see, I'll never be able to understand."

Cornudet spoke up:

"War is barbaric when you attack a peaceful neighbor but it's a sacred duty when you defend the fatherland."

The old woman lowered her head:

"Yes, when you defend yourself, that's one thing; but wouldn't it be better to kill all the rulers who do that kind of thing for their own pleasure?"

Cornudet's eyes flashed:

"Bravo, citizen Follenvie!"

Monsieur Carré-Lamadon was lost in thought. Although he was a fanatical admirer of military heroes, this peasant woman's good sense made him marvel at the wealth that could be created in a nation by the idle who were so costly to it and by labor forces not yet fully exploited, if they were used in the great industrial enterprises that it would take many centuries to complete.

Meanwhile Loiseau left his seat, went to the innkeeper and talked to him quietly. The fat man burst out laughing, coughed and spat out his food; his enormous belly leapt with joy at his companion's jokes and he bought six casks of Bordeaux for delivery in the spring, when the Prussians would be gone.

As soon as they finished supper, they all went to bed, dead-tired.

But Loiseau, who had been very observant, put his wife to bed, then glued his eye, and occasionally his ear, to the keyhole in order to observe what he called "the mysteries of the corridor."

After watching and listening for about an hour, he heard a rustling, looked quickly and caught a glimpse of Boule de Suif, who looked even plumper in her blue, white-laced cashmere nightgown. She was holding a candle and was headed in the direction of the numbered door at the end of the corridor. But the door next to hers opened as she passed and when she returned in a few minutes Cornudet, in shirtsleeves, was following her. They talked in a whisper, then stoppped. Boule de Suif seemed to be blocking the doorway with considerable energy. Unfortunately, Loiseau couldn't hear what they were saying; but finally, as their voices rose, he was able to make out a few things. Cornudet was being passionately insistent:

"Come, you're a fool; what difference can it make?"

Boule de Suif [125

She seemed indignant and answered:

"No, my friend, there are times when you just don't; and besides, here it would be a disgrace."

He seemed not to understand, and asked why. She got angry and raised her voice a little more:

"Why? Can't you understand why? When there are Prussians in the house, maybe even next door?"

He didn't answer. The patriotic modesty of this whore, who wouldn't give her favors in the proximity of the enemy must have rekindled his failing dignity, for after giving her a quick embrace he quietly tiptoed back to his room.

Loiseau found the scene very exciting; he abandoned the keyhole, did a little jig, put on his nightcap, raised the sheet covering his wife's bony carcass, and woke her with a kiss, murmuring:

"Do you love me, darling?"

Then the whole house fell silent. But soon there arose from somewhere, perhaps the cellar, or even the attic, a monotonous, rhythmic, and powerful snore, a dull prolonged roar, mixed with sounds of a boiler at high pressure. Monsieur Follenvie was sleeping.

They had decided to leave at eight, so they all met in the kitchen the next morning; but the vehicle stood alone in the courtyard, with a roof of snow, no horses, no coachman. They couldn't find him in the stables, the barns, or the coach-houses. The men decided to search the countryside for him and went off. They found themselves in the town square, with the church at one end and, on two sides, one-story houses in which they could see German soldiers. The first one they saw was peeling potatoes. The second, a little farther up, was washing the barber-shop floor. Another, whose beard covered his whole face, had his arms around a little boy who was in tears, and rocked him on his knees to stop his crying; and the fat peasant women whose men were all "off to war" showed their conquerors the work to be done in sign language: cut wood, pour the soup on the bread, grind the coffee; one of them was doing the wash for his hostess, an old cripple.

The Count, who was surprised at what he saw, questioned the beadle as he came out of the rectory. The old church-rat answered:

"Oh, they're not bad; not even Prussians, according to what I've heard. They come from farther away, don't know where; and they've all left a wife and children back home; and they don't like war very much, you know. I'll bet their wives are crying for them too; and it'll all make a whole lot of misery for them as well as for us. We're still not too badly off here, because they're not bothering us and they're working as if they were still home. You see, sir, little people have to help each other. . . . It's the big fish who start wars."

Cornudet, who was indignant at this *entente cordiale* between conquerors and conquered, withdrew, preferring to shut himself up in the inn. Loiseau said jokingly:

"They're going to re-populate the country." But Monsieur Carré-Lamadon answered solemnly:

"They're trying to make amends." In any case, the coachman couldn't be found. Finally they found him in the village café, fraternizing with the officer's orderly.

"Weren't you told to have the coach ready at eight?"

"Yes, of course, but I got another order afterwards."

"Namely?"

"Not to harness."

"Who gave you the order?"

"The commandant, by God."

"Why?"

"I have no idea. Go ask him yourself. They tell me not to harness, I don't harness. That's all."

"Did he give you the order himself?"

"No Sir, the innkeeper brought me the message."

"When was that?"

"Last night, when I went to bed."

The three men returned to the inn very upset.

They asked for Monsieur Follenvie, but the servant said that because of his asthma he never got up before ten. He had forbidden her to wake him earlier unless there was a fire.

They asked to see the officer, but that turned out to be absolutely impossible, even though he was quartered at the inn; only Monsieur Follenvie had permission to talk to him about civil affairs. So they waited. The women went to their rooms and passed the time on trifles.

Cornudet made himself comfortable in front of the enormous kitchen fireplace and enjoyed the warmth of the blaze. He had a small table brought to him, ordered a beer, and puffed on his pipe, which was as esteemed among his republican friends as he was, as if by serving his pleasure, it also served the nation. It was a superb meerschaum pipe, beautifully seasoned, black as its owner's teeth, but fragrant, delicately curved, shiny, and familiar to his grip; it was a part of his physiognomy. He sat quite still, staring at the flames or at the foam that crowned his beer-mug; each time he took a drink of the beer he ran his long thin fingers through his greasy hair contentedly and sniffed at his moustache, which was covered with foam.

Loiseau, pretending to go out to stretch his legs, instead visited the local wine-dealers and made a number of sales. The Count and the manufacturer began to talk politics. The Count still believed in the royal family of Orléans, Monsier Carré-Lamadon, in some unknown savior, a hero who would appear when all hope for France was lost, like Du Guesclin, or Joan of Arc perhaps. Or another Napoleon I. Oh, if only the crown prince were not so young! Cornudet overheard them and smiled; he knew what the future held in store for them. His pipe made the kitchen fragrant.

Monsieur Follenvie appeared as it struck ten. They immediately questioned him but he could only repeat over and over again, without changing a word: "This is what the commandant said: 'Monsieur Follenvie, you will not allow these travellers' horses to be harnessed tomorrow. They may not leave without my express order. Do you understand?' That's all."

They tried to see the commandant. The Count sent his card, on which Monsieur Carré-Lamadon wrote his name and titles. The Prussian sent back word that he would receive the two men when he finished breakfast, at around one.

The ladies came down and had a bite to eat despite their concern. Boule de Suif looked ill and troubled.

They were finishing their coffee when the orderly came for the two gentlemen.

Loiseau joined them; but although they tried to persuade Cornudet to come along to give greater solemnity to their delegation, he proudly declared that he would never have anything to do with the Germans, sat down again before the fireplace and ordered another beer.

The three men went up and were ushered into the finest room in the inn, where the commandant received them, finally, stretched out in an armchair, his feet on the hearthstone, smoking a long porcelain pipe probably stolen from an abandoned house owned by a bourgeois with bad taste. He didn't get up, didn't greet them, didn't even look at them. It was a magnificent expression of rudeness that comes naturally to victorious soldiers.

After a few moments he finally said: "What do you want?"

The Count decided to be their spokesman: "We would like to leave, Sir."

"No."

"May we ask why you refuse to allow us to leave?"

"Because I don't want you to leave."

"May I respectfully point out, Sir, that your commanding general signed our pass for Dieppe; and I don't think we've done anything to deserve this harsh treatment."

"I do not want you to leave. . . . That is all. You may go now."

The three men bowed and left.

They spent a wretched afternoon. No one could understand this German capriciousness; the most extraordinary ideas went through their heads. Everyone stayed in the kitchen and debated the matter endlessly, imagining the most outlandish things. Maybe they were to be kept as hostages—but why?—or be taken prisoner? Or most probably they were going to ask for a large ransom? They were panic-stricken at the thought of ransom. The richest ones were the most frightened; they could already see themselves forced to hand over sacks of gold to this insolent soldier to save their lives. They racked their brains to find acceptable lies, to find a way of disguising their wealth or of passing themselves off as poor folk. Loiseau took off his watch-chain and hid it in his pocket. Nightfall made them even more fearful. A lamp was lit, and as they still had two hours before dinner, Madame Loiseau suggested a game of *Trente et Un.* It would get their minds off things. They agreed. Even Cornudet politely put out his pipe and played.

The Count shuffled, dealt, and Boule de Suif won the first hand straight off; very soon the interest they had in the game calmed their obsessive fears. But Cornudet noticed that Loiseau and his wife were both cheating.

As they were about to sit down to table Monsieur Follenvie reappeared and in his gravelly voice announced: "The Prussian officer wishes to know if Mademoiselle Elisabeth Rousset has changed her mind."

Boule de Suif remained standing, white with fury; then turning red all at once she had a fit of choking rage that made it impossible for her to speak. She finally exploded: "Tell that scum, that bastard, that Prussian swine, that I *never* will. Do you understand? Never, never, never!"

The fat innkeeper left. Boule de Suif was quickly surrounded by her companions and questioned; they begged her to reveal the mystery of her visit to the officer. At first she resisted but finally her fury got the best of her: "What does he want? . . . Do you really want to know? He wants to go to bed with me!" she shouted. Their indignation was so violent that no one was offended by her language. Cornudet slammed his beer-mug against the table, cracking it. There were shouts of disapproval of this vicious ruffian, an outcry of collective anger, and a feeling of solidarity and resistance arose among them, as if each had been asked to share the sacrifice demanded of her. In disgust the Count declared that "those people" were behaving like barbarians. The women were especially solicitous of Boule de Suif in their warm and affectionate compassion. The nuns, who showed up only for meals, looked down and said nothing.

They had dinner, nevertheless, once their first outburst of rage had subsided; but there was little talk and much reflection.

The ladies went to bed early; the men sat down for a smoke and decided to play a hand of *Ecarté*; they invited Monsieur Follenvie with the intention of questioning him carefully to determine the best way to overcome the officer's resistance. But he wouldn't take his attention away from his cards and kept repeating: "Play, gentlemen, play." He was so absorbed in his hand that he forgot to spit, which occasionally made his chest give out sounds like organ stops. His wheezing lungs ran the whole asthmatic gamut, from deep base notes to the shrill notes of young cocks trying to crow.

Monsieur Follenvie even refused to go to bed when his wife, who was exhausted, came to get him. So she went up alone; she was an "early-bird," always got up at dawn, while her husband was a "night-owl," always willing to stay up the whole night with friends.

"Don't forget to warm up my eggnog," he shouted, and went back to his game. When it became obvious that they weren't about to get anything out of him, they all agreed that it was time to stop, and so they went to bed.

They got up early again the next morning with a feeling of vague hope, an even greater yearning to get away, and an absolute terror at the thought of spending another day at that wretched little inn.

But, alas! the horses stayed in the stable, the coachman was not to be seen. For want of something better to do they walked around the coach.

Lunch was a melancholy affair. They were visibly less sympathetic toward Boule de Suif now, for during the night, which always brings better judgment, they had somewhat changed their opinion. Now they seemed to be an-

noyed with this girl for not having secretly spent the night
with the Prussian so she could give her companions a pleasant surprise in the morning. Nothing would have been
simpler. And who would have known, after all? She could
have saved face by telling the officer that she was doing it
out of pity for them. And besides, it was such a trifle for
her!

But no one was willing to admit these thoughts yet.

That afternoon they were dying of boredom when the
Count proposed a walk around the village. Everyone
dressed warmly and the little group went off, with the exception of Cornudet, who preferred the warmth of the fire,
and the two nuns, who spent their days either in church or
at the rectory.

The increasingly intense cold stung their noses and
ears; their feet hurt so much that every step was painful
effort; and when the countryside spread out before them
it looked so frightfully dismal under the endless blanket of
snow that they all turned back immediately, depressed and
numb of spirit.

The four women walked ahead, the men followed, a few
steps behind.

Loiseau, who understood how they all felt, wondered
aloud if that "slut" would force them to stay in such a place
much longer. The Count remained courtly; he said no one
could force a woman to make such a painful sacrifice and
it had to come of her own free will. Monsieur Carré-
Lamadon pointed out that if the French counterattacked
from Dieppe the battle would most likely take place near
Tôtes. This worried the others. "What do you think of
escaping on foot?" said Loiseau. The Count shrugged:
"Can you imagine, in this snow? And with our wives? Besides, we'd be followed and caught in ten minutes and
prisoners at the mercy of our captors." He was right; they
fell silent.

The ladies talked about fashions, but a feeling of tension
had come between them.

Suddenly the officer appeared at the end of the street. His wasp-waist was silhouetted against the snow on the horizon and he walked with his legs slightly spread in the manner of soldiers who try to keep their carefully polished boots clean.

He bowed to the ladies as he passed and looked scornfully at the men, who had enough self-respect, moreover, not to tip their hats—though Loiseau made as if to take his off.

Boule de Suif blushed to her ears and the three married women felt humiliated at being seen by the soldier in the company of the woman he had treated so cavalierly.

Talk turned to him, his soldierly bearing, his looks. Madame Carré-Lamadon, who had known many officers and had the judgment of a connoisseur, didn't find him bad at all; she was even sorry he wasn't French, because he would undoubtedly have made a pretty Hussard and women would certainly have lost their heads over him.

They found themselves at loose ends when they got back. They quarreled over trifles. The silent dinner lasted only a few moments and everyone returned to his room, hoping to sleep away the time.

They came down the next morning irritable. The women barely spoke to Boule de Suif.

Church-bells rang for a baptism. The fat girl had a child who was being brought up by peasants in Yvetot. She didn't see him more than once a year and scarcely ever thought of him; but the thought of the child about to be baptized filled her heart with unexpected and deep tenderness for her son and she decided she had to attend the ceremony.

She had no sooner left than they turned to one another and drew up chairs to talk, for they felt that finally something had to be done. Loiseau had an inspiration: they should tell the officer to keep Boule de Suif and let the rest leave.

Monsieur Follenvie was delegated once again for the task, but he came down almost immediately. The German, who understood human nature, had thrown him out. He would keep everybody there until his desire was satisfied.

At that point Madame Loiseau revealed her plebeian nature: "We are *not* going to die here of old age if we can help it. Since it's that tramp's profession to sleep with men, I see no reason why she sould be so particular. She took on anything that came along in Rouen, even coachmen! Yes, Madame, even coachmen, the Prefect's coachman, for example. I know, because he buys our wine. And now that she has a chance to get us out of a mess, this snot-nose plays the virtuous virgin! . . . I think the officer has behaved like a gentleman. Maybe he feels deprived. Besides, I'm sure he would have preferred one of us three. But no, he's perfectly satisfied with a girl who sleeps with anybody. He respects married women. Think for a moment: we are in his power. All he had to say was: 'I want *you*,' and he and his troops would have taken us by force."

The two women shuddered. Madame Carré-Lamadon's eyes shone, and she paled as if she were being raped by the officer.

The men, who had been talking things over by themselves, came up to them. Loiseau was in a rage and wanted to hand over the "little wretch" to the enemy bound hand and foot. But the Count, descended from three generations of ambassadors, and blessed with the looks of a diplomat, preferred the skill of negotiation: "We've got to convince her," he said.

So they began to lay their plan.

The women drew closer, they lowered their voices, and in the ensuing discussion they all gave their opinion as to what they should do. Everything was put in very proper terms. The ladies were most clever in their use of euphemisms and charming and subtle expressions to express the most scabrous things. They observed the niceties of language so carefully that a stranger wouldn't have understood a thing. But the thin layer of propriety that masks ladies of the world is easily removed; they revelled in this indecent adventure, they were really enjoying it enormously; they felt themselves in their true element, marketing love with the sensuality of a cook preparing someone else's supper.

This affair was really so funny to them that their gaiety was quickly revived. The Count made a few slightly risqué remarks, so well turned that they couldn't help provoke smiles. Then Loiseau made a few bolder jokes, but no one took offense; and the thought expressed so brutally by his wife dominated their minds: "Since it's that tramp's profession to sleep with men, I see no reason why she should be so particular." Nice little Madame Carré-Lamadon seemed even to think that in her place she would refuse him less than another.

So they very carefully planned their siege, as if they had a surrounded fortress before them. Everyone agreed on his role, on the arguments to be used, the maneuvers to be executed by each. They established their tactics, their feints, the surprise attacks they would use to force the surrender of this living citadel.

Cornudet, however, stood apart, a stranger to the plot.

They were so completely absorbed that they didn't hear Boule de Suif come back in. But the Count gave a low "Shhh," which made them all look up. She was there. There was a sudden silence and for a few moments their discomfort prevented them from speaking to her. The Countess, more adept at drawing-room hypocrisy than the others, asked: "Did you enjoy the baptism?"

The fat girl, who could still feel the emotion of the ceremony, described everything, the people's faces, the poses they struck, even what the church looked like. She added: "It's so good to pray."

Until lunch-time the ladies were pleased to be friendly to her, to build up her trust in them and her willingness to follow their advice.

As soon as they were all seated they began their approach. They started with a general conversation on self-sacrifice, citing examples from antiquity: Judith and Holophernes, then, irrelevantly, Lucretia and Sextus, and Cleopatra, who took all the enemy generals to bed with her and reduced them to cringing slaves. Then they unfolded an improbable tale, hatched in the imagination of these ignorant millionaires, about the Roman woman who went to Capua and seduced Hannibal and his officers, together with their phalanxes of mercenaries. They cited all the women in history who outwitted the conquerors, used their bodies as battlefields, instruments of victory, weapons, women who overcame hateful monsters with their caresses and sacrificed their chastity to vengeance or dedication to their homeland.

They even talked in veiled terms about the noble young Englishwoman who had herself inoculated with a horrible contagious disease so that she could give it to Bonaparte, who was saved miraculously at the moment of the fatal rendezvous by a momentary weakness.

These things were all said in most proper terms and with no particular emphasis, except for an occasional outburst of enthusiasm aimed at inspiring a passion to emulate these heroines.

One would have thought that the only role of women on earth was perpetual self-sacrifice and a continuous surrender to the whims of lecherous warriors.

The two nuns, lost in deep thought, didn't seem to understand what was being said. Boule de Suif was silent.

They let her ponder the matter all afternoon. But instead of saying "Madame" to her, as they had before, they now addressed her as "Mademoiselle," not knowing exactly why, but as if to bring her down one step from the esteem she had gained and to reveal to her how shameful her situation was.

As the soup was being served, Monsieur Follenvie appeared once again and repeated the familiar declaration: "The Prussian officer wishes to know if Mademoiselle Elisabeth Rousset has changed her mind."

Boule de Suif answered curtly: "No."

At dinner the coalition lost ground. Loiseau made a few clumsy remarks. They were racking their brains to find new examples of self-sacrifice and discovered none, when the Countess, surely without premeditation, and probably feeling a vague need to give praise to Religion, asked the older nun what she could tell them about heroic acts of the saints. Now of course many had committed acts that would be crimes in our eyes but the Church forgives with great ease any misdeed committed for the glory of God or for love of neighbor. That was a powerful argument and the Countess exploited it. Then, as if by tacit agreement, or perhaps because of the secret willingness to oblige in which ecclesiastics seem to excel, or perhaps simply as the result of her fortunate and most helpful stupidity, the old nun brought unexpected aid and comfort to the plotters. They thought she was timid but she turned out to be bold, long-winded and passionate. She wasn't bothered by the subtleties of casuistry; her religion was like an iron bar, her faith was unshakable and her conscience free of scruples. She found Abraham's binding of Isaac perfectly natural, for she would have killed both her mother and her father without hesitation if the order had come from above; and in her opinion nothing could displease the good Lord if the intention was praiseworthy. The Countess, putting the sacred authority of this unexpected accomplice to immediate good use, extracted from the old nun an edifying paraphrase of the moral maxim: "The end justifies the means."

She asked:

"Then you believe, Sister, that God will accept any means, pardon any act, if the motives are pure?"

"How could anyone doubt that for a second, Madame? A reprehensible act is often meritorious because of the thought that inspires it."

And they went on like this, unraveling God's will, foreseeing His judgments, showing Him to be interested in things that were really of little concern to Him.

This was all said indirectly, discreetly, cunningly. But every word the wimpled nun uttered tore a hole in the wall of resistance the indignant courtesan had built. Then the conversation shifted, and the lady of the pendant rosaries talked about her Order, her Mother Superior, about herself and her darling companion, dear Sister St. Nicephora. They had been summoned to Le Havre to take care of hundreds of hospitalized soldiers suffering from smallpox. She described the poor wretches and their symptoms. And to think, she said, that because of this Prussian's whim many Frenchmen whom she and her companion might have saved were going to die! Her specialty was the care of soldiers; she'd been in the Crimea, Italy, Austria, and as she described her military campaigns she became the picture of a warrior nun, the kind who seem born to be camp-followers, pick up the wounded in the swirl of battle, and who can subdue hardened old troopers better than their officers can; a real zealot of a nun whose scarred face, strewn with an infinite number of holes, incarnated the destructiveness of war.

After she spoke there was total silence; she seemed to have done the trick.

When they finished eating they went to bed quickly and came down late the next morning.

Lunch was tranquil by comparison. They wanted to let the seeds they had sown the evening before germinate and bear fruit.

The Countess proposed a walk that afternoon. As agreed, the Count took Boule de Suif by the arm and walked with her, staying a little behind the others.

He talked to her in the familiar, paternal, slightly contemptuous manner gentlemen of distinction use with prostitutes, calling her "ma chère enfant," looking down on her from the height of his social position and indisputable rank. He immediately went to the heart of the matter:

"So, you would rather leave us here, exposed just like you, to the violence that might follow the defeat of the Prussians; you would risk that rather than grant your favors to a man as you have so often in the past?"

Boule de Suif didn't answer.

He then tried to reason with her, cajole her, he played on her feelings. He was able to remain "His Lordship" and to play the gallant, both flattering and familiar, when necessary. He praised the service she would render them, spoke of their gratitude; then, suddenly, gaily switching to the *thou* form of address:

"And you know, my dear, he could boast of having enjoyed the favors of the prettiest girl in the region."

Boule de Suif said nothing, but rejoined the company. When she returned to the inn she went to her room and didn't come down again. They were extremely uneasy. They wondered what she would do. What a dilemma if she said no!

Dinner-time came; still no Boule de Suif. Monsieur Follenvie entered and said that since she was, it seemed, indisposed, they should go ahead. They pricked up their ears. The Count approached the innkeeper and whispered: "Has she made up her mind?"—"Yes." For the sake of propriety, he said nothing to his companions, merely nodding. They immediately breathed a sigh of relief, and their spirits rose. Loiseau cried out: "By Jove, I'll stand champagne for one and all if any can be found in the house," and Madame Loiseau winced when the proprietor came back with four bottles in his hands. They all began to chirp and chatter; joyous gaiety filled their hearts. The Count suddenly realized that Madame Carré-Lamadon was charming; the manufacturer complimented the Countess. The conversation was lively, playful, and witty.

Suddenly, Loiseau, an anxious expression on his face, raised his arms and yelled: "Quiet!" Everyone fell silent, surprised, almost frightened. He cocked his head, silenced them with his two hands, looked at the ceiling, listened again, and continued in a normal voice: "You can set your minds at rest; all's well."

They pretended not to understand; their smiles said otherwise.

Fifteen minutes later, he played the same little game, repeated it numerous times during the evening; he made believe he was speaking to someone on the next floor, giving advice and sprinkling his instruction with *double entendres* from his travelling salesman wit. Occasionally he would sigh sadly: "Poor girl." Or mutter angrily: "You

stinking Prussian." He would take them by surprise by crying out over and over again: "Enough! Enough! Enough!"
And he would add, as if he were talking to himself: "I hope
we'll see her again; he had better not kill her, the ruffian!"

Even though these jokes were in frightful taste, they
were found amusing and no one took offense, for indignation, like everything else, depends on the milieu, and the
atmosphere that had gradually built up around them was
filled with licentious thoughts.

At dessert even the ladies were making sly and witty
remarks. Their faces shone; they'd had quite a bit to drink.
The Count, who preserved his air of gravity even in his slips
of behavior, hit on a very successful comparison involving
the end of a winter's exile at the Pole and the joy of ship-
wrecked sailors who see a route southward open up before
them.

At that moment Loiseau, now ecstatic, took the floor
with a champagne glass in his hand: "I drink to our deliver-
ance!" Everyone got to his feet and cheered. Even the two
nuns were persuaded by the ladies to take a sip of the
sparkling wine they had never tasted. They declared it
tasted like carbonated lemonade, but that it really was finer.

Loiseau summed up the situation: "What a shame
there's no piano; we could have had a quadrille."

Cornudet hadn't said a word or even moved; he seemed
lost in his grave thoughts and kept stroking his great beard
angrily as if he were trying to stretch it. Finally, toward
midnight, as they were about to part company, Loiseau
lurched over to him drunkenly, gave him a pat on the belly,
and burbled: "You're not in a very good mood tonight;
aren't you going to say something, Citizen Cornudet?"
Cornudet jerked his head up and gave them all a flashing
and terrible look: "I tell you you've just done something
infamous!" He got up, went to the door, repeated:
"Infamous!" And disappeared.

For a moment their enthusiasm waned. Loiseau, taken
aback, could think of nothing to answer, then got back his
aplomb: "Sour grapes, old chap, sour grapes." Since they

obviously didn't understand, he explained the "mysteries of the corridor." At which there was another explosion of hilarity. The Count and Monsieur Carré-Lamadon doubled up with laughter. They couldn't believe their ears.

"What! You're sure? He wanted to . . . "

"I tell you I saw him with my own eyes."

"And she refused . . . "

"Because the Prussian was in the next room."

"Impossible."

"I swear it."

The Count nearly choked with laughter. The industrialist held in his sides. Loiseau went on:

"And you can understand why he doesn't think she's very funny tonight, not at all."

They burst out laughing again, coughing, choking, almost apoplectic.

They went their separate ways. But Madame Loiseau, who had the nature of a stinging nettle, pointed out to her husband as they were getting into bed that "that hypocritical little prude" Madame Carré-Lamadon had laughed on the wrong side of her face all evening: "You know, when women have a thing for uniforms, it doesn't make any difference who wears them, Frenchmen or Prussians. Good Lord, what a shame."

All night long in the dark corridor one could hear rustling, barely audible sounds, the padding of bare feet, muted creaks. They got to sleep very late, for streaks of light could be seen under their doors for a long time. Champagne has that effect; it gives you troubled sleep.

The next morning the snow shone under a bright winter sun. The horses were finally harnessed and the coach was waiting before the door; an army of white pigeons with black-dotted pink eyes and puffed-up feathers walked about solemnly between the legs of the six horses and looked for their life's nourishment in the smoking horse-dung they scattered about.

The coachman, huddled in his sheepskin, smoked his pipe as he sat waiting, and all the travellers, beaming, were busy wrapping up provisions for the rest of the trip.

Only Boule de Suif was missing. She came.

She looked a little uncomfortable and ashamed; she moved timidly toward her companions, but they all turned their backs to her as if they hadn't seen her. The Count took his wife's arm with great dignity and took her a safe distance away from this impurity.

The fat girl stopped, not believing her eyes; then, summoning up all her courage, she went up to the manufacturer's wife with a humble "Good morning, Madame." The latter responded with a rude little nod and a look of outraged virtue. Everyone seemed to be very busy, and they kept their distance from her as if she might be carrying a communicable disease in her skirts. Then they rushed into the coach, which she entered last and alone, taking once again the seat she had occupied during the first lap of the trip.

They seemed not to know her, or even see her; but Madame Loiseau, looking at her indignantly, said to her husband in a mock-whisper: "Thank God I'm not sitting next to her."

The massive vehicle started off and the voyage began again.

Not a word was said at first. Boule de Suif didn't dare look up. She felt indignant at her companions, humiliated for having given in, soiled by the kisses and caresses of the Prussian into whose arms they had hypocritically thrown her.

But the Countess, turning to Madame Carré-Lamadon, soon broke the pained silence.

"You know Madame d'Etrelles, don't you?"

"Why yes, she's a friend."

"What a charming woman!"

"Delightful! A really superior woman, well-educated, and an artist to her fingertips; she sings beautifully and draws to perfection."

The manufacturer chatted with the Count, and above the clatter of the windows a word or two could be made out: "Coupons—Maturity—Put and Call—Futures."

Loiseau, who had stolen the worn deck of cards at the inn, cards greasy from being rubbed against dirty tables, started a game of *Bézique* with his wife.

The nuns took their long rosaries from their waists and crossed themselves; and suddenly their lips began to move rapidly, going faster and faster, racing precipitously through their prayers; from time to time they kissed their medals, then crossed themselves again and resumed their rapid and continuous mumbling.

Cornudet sat motionless, thinking.

After about three hours on the road Loiseau picked up his cards: "It's feeding time," he said.

His wife reached for one of the packets of food tied up with string and took out a piece of cold meat. She cut it up neatly into thin but firm slices and the two began to eat.

"We might as well eat too," said the Countess. They all agreed and so she unwrapped the food that had been prepared for the two couples. In one of those long oval dishes the cover of which has a pottery handle in the shape of a hare, to indicate its contents, there was a variety of delicacies; rivers of fat ran around the dark meats of game mixed with other finely chopped meats. There was also a fine square of Gruyère, which had been wrapped in a piece of newspaper and still bore the words "News Items" on its oily surface.

The two nuns unwrapped a piece of garlic sausage; Cornudet plunged both hands into the vast pockets of his greatcoat, taking four hard-boiled eggs out of one and a piece of bread out of the other. He peeled the shells, threw them on the hay beneath his feet, and bit into the eggs, dropping little pieces of yolk on his vast beard, where they shone like stars.

Boule de Suif, who had gotten up in such haste and confusion that she hadn't been able to think of anything, watched them, exasperated and choking down her rage, as they nonchalantly ate. A violent fit of anger made her stiffen and she opened her mouth to cry out what she thought of them with a flood of insults that rose to her lips, but she was paralyzed by her anger.

No one gave her a thought or even looked at her. She felt as if she were drowning in the contempt of these proper scoundrels who had first sacrificed her, then rejected her like an unclean and useless object. Then she thought of her own big basket full of delicacies they had gluttonously devoured, the two chickens, the pâtés, the pears, the four bottles of Bordeaux; suddenly her rage subsided and fell, like the snapping of a tightly drawn rope, and she felt on the verge of tears. She tried desperately to control herself, straightened, swallowed her sobs, like a child; but the tears came, gleaming on her eyelids, and soon two big teardrops dropped from her eyes and rolled gently down her cheeks. Others followed, faster, flowing like drops of water that seep through a crack in a stone, falling rhythmically on the full roundness of her breasts. She sat straight up, hoping they wouldn't see her.

But the Countess noticed her crying and nudged her husband. He shrugged as if to say: "What can I do? It's not my fault." Madame Loiseau chuckled triumphantly and murmured: "Tears of shame."

The two nuns had started praying again after wrapping up the rest of their sausage.

Then Cornudet, who was contentedly digesting his eggs, stretched out his legs under the seat, lay back, crossed his arms, and, like someone who has just witnessed a very funny scene, began to whistle the "Marseillaise."

At the sound of the anthem there were angry looks.

His companions were not pleased by the sound of the revolutionary song. They became restless and irritated and seemed to be ready to howl as dogs do when they hear a hand-organ. He noticed their annoyance and went right on. Occasionally he would even hum the words:

> *Amour sacré de la patrie*
> *Conduis, soutiens nos bras vengeurs,*
> *Liberté, liberté chérie,*
> *Combats avec tes défenseurs!*

The colder the snow got, the faster the horses went; and right up to Dieppe, during the long morning hours, over the endless bumps in the road, through the darkening evening, then in the totally obscure interior when night fell he kept up his monotonous but vengeful whistling with ferocious insistence, forcing their tired and irritated minds to follow the song from beginning to end and making them remember each and every word and beat.

And Boule de Suif cried; sometimes an uncontrollable sob would make its way into the darkness between two lines of the "Marseillaise."

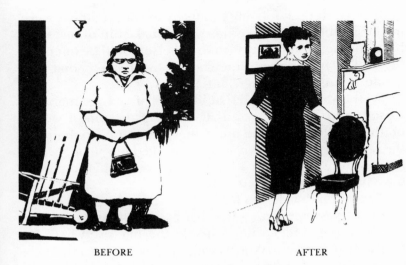

BEFORE   AFTER

LEONA WAS THE BUTTERBALL AT THANKSGIVING UNTIL SHE TRIED OUR DIET PLAN

I came from a big farm family, and we always liked to spend a lot of time sitting around the table after dinner. Except everybody else would be talking and drinking coffee, while I went around finishing off the pies and sneaking all the scraps I could find!

From the time I was a little bitsa thing I was always bigger than the other kids, Mama used to say it was baby fat, but it took half a dozen scrambled eggs and half a loaf of bread to get me going in the mornings, and that was only the beginning! Rich desserts, meat loaf sandwiches in front

145

of the TV after school, doughnuts by the dozen, those were my meat, and if the other kids would make fun of me, why, have another doughnut! Everybody else would be out playing ball or helping with the chores, but Little Leona, she would be inside with her "little snack."

Well I wasn't really all that big until after I got married, I used to go to parties and all, but half the time I would be the wallflower by the punchbowl, eating everything on the table. Ken didn't care, he said he liked big strong women, he said "I do" with a big smile, even though my wedding dress was a tight size 20!

Then Ken decided to leave the farm and he moved me and Lisa (yes there was a new baby—and 30 extra pounds on me!) to a trailer camp outside the big city where he found factory work. Well I was lonesome and homesick, and on top of that there was going to be another baby, so I just stayed in the trailer and ate and ate!

Ken was so sweet he never said anything, and I used to kid myself after Bubba came, I would stay away from mirrors and wear my old maternity clothes until even those got too tight. Then I would buy those big old flowered tents in the old ladies' departments, I didn't even want to know what size they were. I was only 23 but I looked 55 years old! Oh, I tried to diet, but it was a drop in the bucket, so I stopped.

Well after a couple of years of Ken working round the clock and babies crying and me eating, we packed up and went home to the farm. I couldn't figure out why Ken was embarrassed until we went to the first big party, the first Thanksgiving dinner since we got home.

Oh they were all polite, but Ken's niece Lena was too little to know any better, so when somebody told Ken's mother the turkey was real good and she said it was a Butterball, I heard Lena piping up: I'll tell you who's the butterball! They all shushed her but everybody was looking at me. I could have died right there!

Well I went home and cried and cried and cried, Ken said don't mind them but I said maybe they're right, and then he wouldn't look at me so I knew. I wanted to die but I saw your ad in a magazine and I thought maybe there is hope. I've been on your diet plan for 18 months now. I've come down from those huge tents to a trim size 14 and I'm aiming for 12 by Christmas.

Ken is so proud of me, I have lots of nifty clothes and even Little Lena calls me Aunt Glamorpuss now that I've trimmed down. Now the only Butterball around our house is on the table! You too can be a glamorpuss, all you have to do is fill in the coupon and send it to the address below. No matter how fat you are, you too can lead a new life.

(Advertisement)

FAT GIRL

by *Brendan Gill*

JEANNE was a big, soft bolster of a girl, with no sharp edges anywhere. She had sky-blue eyes that would suddenly go blank and, after a few seconds, as suddenly come back into focus, and if this was strange what was stranger still was the fact that she seemed to be unaware that it was happening. There was also something odd about her pouting mouthful of pearly teeth—either they were exceptionally small and fine or, young as she was, they were false. Her feet were broad and flat-soled, and from a long way off she could be heard marching slump-slump over the linoleum-covered floors of the office corridors. She had a pretty face, with a well-modelled nose and a high, smooth forehead, from which her hair was drawn back in fine, light-gold threads to a bun behind. Men fell in love with her readily, and she was not surprised.

Two years ago, at eighteen, Jeanne got her first full-time job, with a firm of engineers in a building in the East Forties. The firm is a large one, occupying several floors in the tower of the building; from the office windows you look far out over Long Island, whose distant reaches seem an unpeopled low green wilderness against the sky. Until early this summer, when a number of substantial aircraft contracts were cancelled, the firm had enjoyed many years of unbroken prosperity. At the first hint of hard times, it started cutting down on its office staff, and Jeanne was certain to be among those who would be dismissed, more because her dismissal would serve as a warning to other

girls on Jeanne's secretarial level that they must henceforth
work harder than they were used to than because the firm
was in serious financial difficulties. "We are taking advantage of this opportunity of putting our house in order," the
president of the firm noted, not without relish, in a memo-
randum circulated among his board of directors. "A little
bad news can be a healthy thing."

A week or so later, on the very day that Jeanne was given
notice, she was battered to death by a young photographer
with whom she had been living. (Though the newspapers
didn't mention it, an executive of the firm was with her at
the time. Roused by her screams, he ran to get help from
neighbors, and so may have escaped being murdered himself.) Jeanne's death was shocking for many reasons, not
the least of which was the discovery that she had, or appeared to have, no family. The data she had given the
personnel office on applying for a job—place of birth, parents, schooling, and the like—had all been made up, perhaps on the spur of the moment. In any event, the body
was never claimed by relatives, and after the police were
finished with it it was buried, without a funeral ceremony,
in the plot of a family named Archer, in a small cemetery
in Connecticut.

People in the office found it incomprehensible that
good-natured, slow-moving, slovenly Jeanne could be im-
plicated in a deed so violent and bloody—the weapon the
young man used in smashing her skull was a camera tripod,
and it did its work badly—but the fact is that her fate was
in every way characteristic of her; she died as she did because, up to the very last moment of her life, she was kind,
lazy, and accommodating; a fat girl content with her lot,
who pleased herself and pleased others.

The two most extraordinary things about Jeanne were
her size and her skin, which didn't resemble ordinary human skin at all; it was as if she had been upholstered in yard
upon yard of some marvellous translucent fabric, very thin
and strong, which had been drawn taut over her abundant
flesh and blood and which effortlessly kept in place the

clutter of her internal organs. When that silky pinkness was touched anywhere, it went white, then red, and the mark of fingers remained on the spot for a long while afterward. A stranger taking hold of her nakedness with his eyes closed might have supposed that he had come into possession of a bundle of some ancient, sumptuous Venetian bedding, and he would have been every bit as astonished when, from time to time, the bedding stirred of its own accord or gave up a sleepy sigh, as when, at the very start of lovemaking, a small, pointed tongue emerged from the pale, little-girl lips and set conscientiously to work.

What puzzled everyone at first was not only her size but also her attitude toward her size, which was one of unquestioning approval. She was totally unlike most fat girls, who suffer openly or secretly from their condition; they rarely choose, as Jeanne did, to ignore the problem. More accurately, not "ignore," since for her the problem didn't exist; her body satisfied her just as it was, and if, undressing her in your mind, your lust was given a momentary check by the thought of the thickness of the great thighs guarding the portal of her trunk, or by the thought of the loop of flesh that would surely hang from her waist as she knelt swaying above you in bed, it was, Jeanne seemed to imply, your loss, not hers—let your goggle-eyed adolescent mind busy itself undressing other girls, the skinnier the better. She managed to convey without the least taint of vanity the impression that she believed herself to be a remarkable physical specimen. It was as if she had gathered up every scrap of available information about herself and had fed it into a computer and had then learned, without surprise, that the reading provided by the computer was the single word "Perfect."

Jeanne took exceptional pleasure in eating and drinking. They were activities that she engaged in aggressively, as other people climbed mountains or competed in games. The sight of food and liquor made her eyes shine. Her first meal of the day was a hasty one—so hasty that she often had no recollection of having eaten it and would say later to girls in the office that it was no wonder she felt starved, having had to go without breakfast that morning. It was her own fault that the meal had to be gobbled on the run. She set her alarm clock to go off too late to allow time for all the tasks she knew she ought to perform in the apartment; moreover, when the alarm rang, she frequently turned it off without so much as opening her eyes and, hugging a pillow in her big bare arms, dozed until the second warning system, a clock-radio on the bureau well beyond her reach, filled the room with its clangor. Jeanne would then plunge groaning up out of bed, a cloud of pink skin that smelled of a childish intensity of sleep and, ever so faintly, of the previous evening's cigarettes and whiskey, and stumble through washing and dressing. In that morning rush, it was impossible for her to leave her room as tidy as she hoped to find it on her return. She acted as if she believed in a magic by which inanimate objects would be able to perform their own housekeeping, and the bed that she left unmade in the morning was always a disappointment to her when she came home at night and found it still unmade. As she clumped heavily down the stairs of the apartment house, the taste of breakfast, which consisted of whatever she had managed to find in her closet-sized kitchen—an open Coca-Cola and a couple of brick-hard brownies, say, or, with luck, a leftover hamburger flecked with white grease and all the more delicious for being cold—mingled not unpleasantly in her mouth with the taste of toothpaste and fresh lipstick.

Jeanne was expected to reach the office by nine, but she was always late, in part because she allowed herself too little time to walk the ten or twelve blocks between her apartment house on First Avenue in the Fifties and the office, and in part because she stopped at a delicatessen along the way to pick up a Danish pastry ring and a plastic container of coffee. ("Heavy on the cream," she would say, in her sweet, rather infantile voice.) Reaching the office, she lifted the coffee and pastry out of their brown paper bag and set them on her desk, on a blotter that bore the

stain marks of innumerable other coffee containers of precisely the same circumference. With a concentration that
turned the simple, necessary acts into a ceremony, she
prized the lid off the container of coffee, unwrapped the
waxed paper from around the Danish, and sat motionless
for a few seconds, enjoying the look of the steam that rose
from the coffee and the crisp fragrance of the pastry. She
picked up the ring in both hands, the plump little fingers
held at a sharp angle to the rest, and bit off the ring in large
chunks, working them as steadily into her mouth as if she
were stoking a furnace. Now and again, she would stop to
wipe flakes of pastry from her smeared lips and chin, not
with the paper napkin provided by the delicatessen but with
her fingertips, which she would afterward lick carefully, one
by one. When the Danish was finished and her fingers
thoroughly licked, she ran the palms of her hands along the
sides of her chair, which was covered with a stout brown
furze and which, in the course of her two years in the office,
took on a hard, yellowish patina. She ended by brushing
any remaining crumbs of Danish from her lap onto the
floor and uttering a long-drawn-out sigh of satisfaction.
She fed and cleaned herself with the raptness of some out-
size domestic animal, staring straight ahead of her and
seeing nothing; she didn't like to be spoken to on such
occasions, and despite her good nature she would generally refuse to answer any questions that were put to her,
affecting as a form of politeness not to hear them.

This was the first of several between-meal snacks that
Jeanne treated herself to in the course of the day. The
second came shortly after ten, when Amos Archer, for
whom she worked as secretary, arrived at the office. Archer
would be as breathless as if he had just raced in on foot
from Riverdale, though in fact he lived in a single room in
a cheap hotel across the street. Sometimes it happened that
smoke would be curling up out of the right-hand pocket
of his tweed jacket when he arrived. Archer had old-fash-
ioned good manners and believed that nobody should
smoke in elevators; on entering one he would thrust his

lighted pipe into his pocket and, as often as not, would forget its presence there until somebody happened to notice the smoke, or until the jacket itself, after smoldering away for a time (his jackets were famously old and threadbare and as dry as tinder), would suddenly burst into flames, which Archer would beat out with his bare hands, shouting "Damn! Damn! Damn!" in a high voice that sounded not altogether displeased with his adventure.

Archer was a good-looking, gray-haired man who, in his fifties, gave an impression of benign senility. He let his glasses ride well down over the bridge of his nose, and he would fix his attention on you over the tops of them, perhaps thinking that this would serve to increase the seeming sharpness of his appraisal of you. What it did, on the contrary, was to make him look dimmer and more elderly than ever—a foxy grandpa who had somehow prematurely mislaid his foxiness. Trained as an engineer, he had long since been eased out of any responsibility for design in the firm; though he was listed as one of the vice-presidents, he had been reduced to serving as a sort of office manager, whose duties were supposed to consist of keeping the place in order. It was he who parcelled out the chronically insufficient office space and purchased necessary equipment and supplies, and the high-strung ineffectiveness with which he performed these tasks was, for as long as the office remained prosperous, a cherished office scandal—Archer was the example always cited when the senior partners wished to reassure themselves that, big and rich as the firm had grown, it had not lost the common, cranky touch.

Archer and Jeanne suited each other to perfection. They were alike in geniality and incompetence, and from the start their days passed without friction and without accomplishment. As soon as Archer had seated himself at his desk, Jeanne would hurry down to the short-order restaurant in the lobby of the building and ask for tea and a buttered raisin bran muffin for Archer and a blueberry muffin and coffee for herself. ("Heavy on the cream," she would say again, not for the last time that day.) Scattering crumbs of muffin along his desk and occasionally, with too violent a gesture, overturning his tea—"God damn these silly containers! Why don't they make the bottoms broader than the tops? Why don't they *engineer* them? My under-drawers are soaking!"—he would harangue her passionately from his inner office about the problems heaped on his shoulders by his unconscionable superiors, while Jeanne in the glass-walled outer office would sit munching her muffin and sipping her coffee, hearing nothing and saying nothing.

Once they had finished their snack, Archer would summon her to his desk and set about dictating memoranda, in extended reply to memoranda received by him from other executives of the company. Jeanne had claimed, applying for the job, to be capable of taking shorthand, but this was no doubt as untrue as everything else she had set down on that occasion; she wrote out laboriously, in a round, childish longhand, the messages that Archer intended to have strike like thunderbolts his innumerable adversaries up and down the hall. He spoke rapidly, in bursts of intricately cluttered phrases, and Jeanne would have been unable to set down six consecutive words as he had uttered them, but her incompetence scarcely mattered; no sooner had he tossed off a sentence than it turned out that he was merely testing the sound of it. "No, no, change that, change that!" he would exclaim, with mounting excitement, for the power of veto, even though it was being exercised only against himself, invariably went to his head. "Make it 'In answer to your inquiry'—no, make it 'In answer to your impertinent inquiry'—no, let's save 'impertinent' for later—make it just 'inquiry'—'inquiry of the seventeenth, let me refresh your recollection concerning the disposition of the . . . ah, the desk and chairs that you have the impertinence to imply'—yes, 'impertinence' is excellent there—'the impertinence to imply were promised you as of the first of the month. Nothing could be farther—further?—farther from the truth. Indeed . . .' "

By one, the usual time at which Jeanne went to lunch, she was again, so she claimed, starved. If she was having lunch with some of the girls in the office, they went to the nearest Schrafft's or Stouffer's, but if, as was more likely, she was being taken to lunch by some man in the office, or by some client of the firm whom she had met, this guaranteed a substantial meal at one or another of the three or four middle-priced French restaurants in the neighborhood. In any event, lunch was always preceded by her first drink of the day: a vodka Martini on the rocks. "*Oh,* but that's *good!*" she would protest, in a tone of astonishment, as if she had never tasted alcohol before and had heard nothing but bad about it. Three or four long swigs and her glass would be empty. Most of the other girls, whose masters were sterner than Jeanne's, would limit themselves to a single drink, but Jeanne had no fear of Archer, and the speed with which she gulped the first Martini allowed her ample time for a second before the usual fruit salad or grilled-cheese sandwiches arrived.

When Jeanne was with a man and he asked her if she would like a second drink (his attention having perhaps been called to this possibility by Jeanne's habit of spinning ice cubes about in the empty glass with her forefinger), she would roll her sky-blue eyes and say, "I know I shouldn't, but, oh, Lord . . ." Later, if the man asked whether she would like a glass of wine with her meal, she would roll her eyes again and in the same voice say, "I know I shouldn't, but . . ." And if the man proposed a bottle of wine instead of a glass, Jeanne's spirits would rise in proportion. "That would be *lovely,*" she would say, reaching her hand out over the red-checked tablecloth and giving her companion's hand a warm, prolonged squeeze. The palm of her hand would be moist; by this time her smooth, high forehead would be covered with innumerable tiny beads of sweat. "Mr. Archer will be furious."

"Nonsense. He's dotty over you."

"No. Yes. That's true. He's a lamb."

"Who happens to bark like a dog. Yap, yap, yap."

"No, no, no!"

"Yap!"

"Nope!"

Delighted with their wit, they filled the restaurant with a shout of laughter. Heads turned, regarding them.

When she had lunch with the girls, she was back at the office by two-thirty; when she had lunch with a man she rarely got back before three-thirty and sometimes as late as four. On these exceptionally tardy occasions, Archer would greet her by not greeting her, silence serving him as a sign of wounded feelings, and Jeanne would spend much of the rest of the short afternoon making up to him and forcing him to forgive her. She was, of course, drunk, but less conspicuously so than one might have expected, and, while it was impossible for her to work at anything that required precision (the typewriter keys swam before her eyes in a blur of %'s and @'s), she found a dozen harmless errands to perform between their offices. She would think of questions to ask that required her to seat herself, dishevelled and pinkly incandescent, beside his desk, or she would carry in papers to sign that permitted her to hover beside him, her damp bosom grazing his head, and the bizarrely mingled smells of her body—Johnson's baby powder, Arpège, garlic, cigarette tobacco, and the odor of skin and hair—would steadily, relentlessly encircle him. Soon he would be sputtering away on the subject of the intolerable burden he bore on behalf of the company night and day without a word of complaint to anyone, and Jeanne would perceive that she had been forgiven, not for the first time, not for the last.

Sometime between four and five, depending on the hour of her return from lunch, she would pay a second visit to the restaurant in the lobby, picking up two orders of tea, toast, and strawberry jam, with perhaps a couple of slices of pound cake on the side, or a piece of lemon meringue pie—dishes that she described every day to Archer as "your special surprises." Archer never tasted them; half a piece of toast without jam, dipped into milky tea, was as much as his stomach dared to encounter at that hour. Jeanne would consume the surprises to the last morsel, saying with the coquettish smile that she used only when she spoke of food, "Waste not, want not." She had a large stock of such sayings, which she squandered continuously throughout the day: "A stitch in time saves nine." "Let sleeping dogs lie." "Least said, soonest mended." She used them like stage money, in lieu of the real thing; they let her hold up her end in conversations without the bother of taking thought, and the pleasure she derived from not thinking became a part of her companion's pleasure, as palpable as the touch of her hand or mouth.

Tea over, it was a matter of scarcely an hour before it was time to stop work for the day. Jeanne's mind would have begun to clear by then, which meant that an energetic befuddlement was replaced by torpor. She enjoyed this lull between periods of drinking; as the first waves of a delectable lassitude stole up her legs and into the stronghold of her body, she would march along the hall to the ladies' room and, kicking off her broad, ugly pumps, stretch herself out on the couch that occupied a third of the little, mirrored anteroom. Provided that she had remembered that morning, in the hurried hurly-burly of dressing, to furnish herself with a handkerchief, she would arrange it daintily over as much of her face as it could be made to cover; otherwise, and more commonly, she would cover her face with a couple of pieces of Kleenex, or, failing that, with a few lengths of the cheap speckled white toilet paper that Archer had ordered no telling how many thousands of rolls of over the years. She held the paper in place with her left arm, which she kept crooked over her eyes to shut out the harsh, naked fluorescent light above her in the ceiling, and to any of the girls who happened in before she fell asleep she explained that she was taking forty winks. That was one of her usual sayings—"forty winks." She had never been known to say that she was going to take a nap. As the girls went to and from the toilets and sinks, or stopped in front of the mirror to comb their hair and restore their makeup, they chattered together without regard for the bulky object on the chintz-covered couch behind them. They knew that once Jeanne had fallen asleep, no ordinary sound would waken her. From time to time, she would speak a word aloud, or utter a faint moan, in response to some remembered or perhaps only dreamed-of pleasure; then her enormous thighs would part, her legs separating into the upright strokes of an A and her plump feet, pink toes packed together inside gauzy nylon, pointing stiffly left and right, like the feet of dolls.

The alarm that served to rouse her from her forty winks was the hubbub of closing time, when the door of the ladies' room was in constant, clattering motion. Jeanne uncrooked her arm, removed the handkerchief or paper covering her eyes, and peered at the ceiling unseeing, as, slowly and with difficulty, she came back into the world. She got up, thrusting her feet reluctantly into her pumps, and made her way into the bathroom proper, where she splashed cold water onto her closed eyelids, dried her face and hands with half a dozen paper towels, and returned to the anteroom. She stared fixedly at herself in the mirrored wall, repeating softly, "Oh, God, oh, God." Then she borrowed lipstick and eye-shadow from one or another of the girls, made up her face in slapdash fashion, and walked slump-slump to the office, where Archer, unmindful of the hour, was sure to be hammering away on his ancient typewriter, the room blue with smoke.

Teetering in the doorway: "Time to stop, Mr. Archer."

"Stop now? Stop *now?*" A fusillade on the keys, struck at great speed with two fingers. "Just getting started."

"Tomorrow is another day."

"I like working late, after the rabble has gone. Gives me a chance to use my head."

If she happened to have no date that evening, or if the date was a late one: "Come buy me a drink instead."

"You've already drunk too much today."

"You're not my father."

"Old enough to be. Your grandfather, if I'd got into trouble early enough. You were practically falling down when you got back from lunch. Which of my lecherous, aging colleagues was trying to seduce you, God damn the whole mindless lot of them?"

"Nobody."

"Ha! No kneesies, no invitations to a midtown matinée?"

"Just one drink. Then you can send me home."

"Never. Not a drop."

In the end, they would go across the street to a small bar in the hotel where Archer lived, and he would buy her the one drink that she had exacted from him and in return would try to learn from her something about her relationships not only with the men in the office (this as possible ammunition for his running battle with them) but also with the college boys who were, so he instructed Jeanne, her only suitable beaux. Archer had been married twice and divorced twice and had no children. His idea of how a good father ought to behave toward a daughter like Jeanne—and he never for a moment risked assuming any other role— was based on recollections of how his father had behaved toward him and his sisters forty years earlier. He gave her advice, but he had no confidence in it, and he was grateful that she did not laugh at him. He was also grateful that she spared him, surely as much from boredom as discretion, particulars of her relationships with men. When she spoke about sexual matters, it was in general terms, and with unselfconscious candor. One gathered that she felt about sexual activity much as she did about her body: that it was a good in itself and had, and needed to have, no connection with any emotion of love. She spoke of other people's sexual practices with an ease that astonished men of Archer's age. She seemed to assume that anyone who had the ability to go to bed would do so as often as possible and that the choice of a partner was by no means the crucial aspect of the performance; which was to say that it was, after all, only a performance and could be judged accordingly. Sometimes, when she was having lunch with girls from the office and they happened to be seated near a window giving them a view of the street, she would offer comments on one or another of the male passersby. "That one there, in plaid," she would say. "He'd be great in bed."

"Jeanne, what a faker you are," one of the girls would say, egging her on. "Nobody can tell by looking."

And Jeanne would smile her pearly smile and say, "*I* can."

Four or five evenings a week, Jeanne went out on dates. Her escorts ranged in age from twenty to sixty. The very young men were unmarried, but nearly all of the rest had wives or, at the least, ex-wives. Most of them were commuters, with houses in Westchester or Connecticut, and no doubt their wives were used to eating dinner alone or with the children. Married men in their thirties who took Jeanne out were inclined to be still somewhat uneasy over not catching their habitual trains; to keep their wives from worrying about them, they felt obliged to telephone home that they had been held up in town on business, but they hated to have Jeanne overhear the falsehoods that made it possible for them to be with her—perhaps to be sprawled with her, telephone in hand, on her rumpled couch, with their loafers off and their mouths a smear of lipstick. Sometimes she found the evidence of their discomfiture touching, as when a young man would wait until she went to the bathroom before picking up the phone and, in a low voice, telling his wife in the suburbs the squalid, necessary lie.

Jeanne wondered why the young men took everything so hard. Their bad consciences were a matter of indifference to her, except to the extent that she was puzzled by their having them. What possible injury could be done to anyone, directly or indirectly, by a man's taking her to dinner and, in some cases, to bed? Even if some of them fell in love with her, what harm? She would never try to take them away from their wives; she was neither ambitious enough nor conspiratorial enough to find such an undertaking attractive. She was lazy and she disliked secrets. The guilty feelings of the young men were tiresome, which was one of the many reasons that she preferred going out with older men; they would have solved any problems in respect to the structure of their private lives long before. They liked feeling desire for her, whether they acted on it or not, and they liked having a companion for whom other men obviously felt desire. Finally, they liked her because she made no demands. She was warm and soft and slovenly and cheerful, and these are qualities that young men do not put a sufficient value on.

The youngest of her regular escorts was a black messenger boy in the office, who invariably took her to a mock-Irish pub in the same block as her apartment house and stared at her over baconburgers and beer for a couple of hours, scarcely speaking a word (the jukebox, which he fed continuously, took his place as the object she was expected to listen to, and Jeanne was well satisfied with this arrangement), and the oldest was the senior vice-president of the firm, a celebrated engineer and no less celebrated womanizer, who had had a heart attack a year or so earlier and who was terrified of dying of a second attack. No longer willing to risk making love, he was as eager as ever to be in the presence of desirable girls, and more eager than ever to be *seen* to be in their presence; he would take Jeanne to "21" or Quo Vadis and sit staring at her with something like the same immobile, silent longing as the young black, while Jeanne ate and drank with gusto and from time to time brushed his cheek with her open mouth.

Jeanne lived on the fourth floor of her apartment house. Since it was a walkup, the vice-president was forced, for his heart's sake, to meet and say good night to her in the tiny ground-floor lobby. Most of the other men in the office felt that they owed it to their manhood to make the climb to her door at the beginning and end of the evening, hoping for much or little according to their natures. It was a stiff climb, and when they rang her bell at the top of the third long flight of stairs they would be breathing hard. Some of them, aiming to give an impression of youthful vitality, would wait a minute or two outside her door to catch their breath, but, if Jeanne had ever troubled herself with such trifles, the ruse would not have deceived her at all—they had to press the button beside her name in the vestibule of the lobby in order for her to release the lock of the front door, and she could have calculated to the second how long it would take them to reach her floor. In fact, she had no thoughts about them between the time they pressed the button downstairs and the time they pressed the button outside her door. When she opened the door, they began to exist, and when she closed it they stopped existing: it was as simple as that. If they were visibly winded, she took pity on them, and this was never, as they feared, because she assumed that their momentary fatigue was a sign of diminished sexual power. Her imagination was exceptionally economical; she could entertain a single concern for a long time without feeling obliged to let it lead her into a second or third one. Sometimes, greeting them at her door and, for a wonder, being ready to go out, she would say, "Poor thing, you look exhausted! Don't you want to come in and rest?" And her middle-aged escort, wanting nothing so much as a few minutes' respite in her blowsy living room, would reply pantingly, "Nonsense! Never . . . felt . . . better in my life! Away we go!"

Equally contrary to what Jeanne's admirers supposed was how little she speculated about their bodies. In her presence, the older men fretted to themselves about their approaching or actual baldness, about their jowls and thickening waists, about the bellies that could no longer be sucked in and rendered comparatively invisible. They would hold their heads unnaturally erect to strengthen the line of the jaw, and, seated, they would keep a picture magazine spread on their knees to conceal the flagrant thrust of their pots. At the moment of undressing, they would become as skittish as maidens, turning off lights and taking advantage of half-opened closet doors to hide behind, then making a rush, phantoms of white, rippled, un-

gainly flesh, for her ill-made bed. Jeanne, who undressed
at leisure in the bathroom, would return to find her bedroom in darkness, the man tucked away under the covers
and dimly smiling, like a child in a nursery waiting for
Nanny's good-night kiss. "But I can't *see* anything!" Jeanne
would complain, turning on the light beside the bed and
throwing herself down naked beside the man, with only the
thickness of the covers left between them. Propping herself
up on one elbow, her big body running the length of the
bed like an Appalachian range of translucent pinky-white
alabaster, she would say, "Let me look at you," and throw
back the covers, exposing him. She would contemplate him
without haste, reaching out from time to time to touch his
body at one point or another and saying, to his astonishment and pleasure, "Nice. Oh, that's nice."

Jeanne's agreeable promiscuity, centered for so many
months on the office, was brought to an end when a young
man named Ross Fisher fell in love with her. He was a
graduate student at Columbia, getting a Ph.D. there for his
parents' sake but planning, for his own sake, to become the
greatest photographer in the world. They met at a cocktail
party one weekend, somewhere in the gusty upper reaches
of Riverside Drive, and that was the first thing he ever said
to her: "I'm going to be the greatest photographer in the
world."

"Do you always say that to people when you first meet
them?"

"To girls I do."

"And are they always very impressed?"

"They always say I ought to be analyzed and I always
say I've tried that, so then we take it from there. Or we
don't take it from there, you know."

Afterward, neither of them could remember the name
of their host, or even why they had happened to go to the
party, and Ross considered these facts proof that they had
been ordained to meet. Promptly at five the following Monday, Ross was at the office to pick up Jeanne and take her

to dinner. He was there on Tuesday as well, and on Wednesday; by then, everyone in the office was aware that an intense courtship was under way—indeed, Ross had announced it to the girl at the reception desk. "I'm courting Jeanne," he said. "I'm going to take her by storm, you'll see. Once I make up my mind to do a thing, nothing can stop me."

Even Archer, who seemed to observe so little, soon became aware of Ross. By the end of the first week, he was in the habit of nodding to Ross, and by the end of the second week he occasionally went so far as to utter a muffled "Hi" to him. Working his pipe up and down in his strong yellow teeth, Archer said one morning to Jeanne, "Not much to look at, but at least he's the right age."

"I hate the babies you want me to like."

"Give him a chance."

"He won't let me not. I wonder what makes him so sure I won't get sick of him. I always do, his type."

"That young man seems pretty sure of everything."

Archer had been wrong to say that Ross was not much to look at. He was a slender, small-boned boy, with features that had the look of having been almost too carefully chosen. Because he was the same height as Jeanne, beside her he seemed smaller than he was. It was true, moreover, that he weighed less than she did, which led to a good deal of ribald speculation in the office about the ways and means of their making love. In fact, there was nothing particularly novel about it. Ross had known but two or three girls, and they had been as inexperienced and tentatively exploratory as he. He was enchanted by the speed and ease with which Jeanne engulfed him. It was as if the boundaries of their bodies had been abrogated; there was no beginning or end to him or to her. In whatever fashion, or sequence of fashions, she led their flesh to become entangled, the feeling on his part was always that of being plunged—weightless, his heart bursting—into an abyss. Making love with Jeanne was by far the most extraordinary physical experience of his life, and sitting beside her afterward at a bar, or across from her at some rickety restaurant table, he marvelled at the composure with which, having returned to the world, she faced the world. The tranquil impassivity of that big body had no connection with the fierce engine that had wracked him and wrung him and left him a breathless eunuch, curled in its shadow.

For Jeanne, Ross was a lover like any other. With time, she knew, he would learn to give her greater satisfaction, but what he already gave her was enough for her needs. It was the surprising modesty of these needs that made it easy for her to say that she would try to be faithful to him. At first, it had not occurred to her that this would be a matter of concern to Ross; she was amused and touched by how shocked he was to discover, in the early stages of their affair, that she was continuing to see and go to bed with other men. It turned out that he had not supposed, from what he had read and heard about affairs, that such conduct was permissible. He was still more shocked when, having accused her of behaving unnaturally, she laughed at him. "Unnatural would be *not* going to bed with people I like to go to bed with," Jeanne said.

"I don't want to make love to anyone but you."

"Then you don't have to."

"And I don't want you to make love to anyone but me."

"That's being piggy."

"People who love each other—"

"Oh, Christ! Who said anything about that?"

"You have, in bed."

"Those times don't count. You always beg me to say something then, so I do."

He said furiously, again a six-year-old, "I'll kill you if you go to bed with anyone else."

"Sticks and stones can break my bones, but words will never hurt me."

He burst into tears, and she held him in her arms on the edge of the bed. When he could speak again, he said, "I *am* going to be the greatest photographer in the world, you wait and see. You'll be terribly proud of me."

"If you don't stop that kind of baby talk, I'll never be proud of you."

He curled his fingers into her bare thigh; the skin went white. "That hurt?"

"Yes."

"Now?"

"Yes."

"Want me to stop?"

"I don't give a damn what you do."

"Tell me to stop. Tell me to stop. Tell me to stop."

But she would say nothing. Eventually, he took his hand away, and the red and white mark of his fingers was on her thigh for days.

She had intended not to see him anymore, but she could never stay angry with anyone for long. She not only went on seeing Ross but agreed to make the experiment of remaining faithful to him. The only condition that she exacted for what he solemnly called her "fidelity" was that he never ask whether she was having sex with someone else. There was no way for him to be sure that her fidelity was absolute, but after a few weeks she allowed him to move into her apartment, and this was assurance of a kind: if she was ever with another man, at least it was no longer in the bed that she shared with Ross.

His presence in the apartment proved a convenience to her, as well as a guarantee to him that he enjoyed privileges in respect to her time and body greater than anyone else enjoyed. For it turned out that Ross had a natural bent for housework. He was as tidy in his domestic habits as Jeanne was sloppy in hers. In the morning, it was he who insisted on their making the rumpled bed that Jeanne would have left unmade until evening, and sometimes when, despite his repeated warnings, she was late for work he would hurry her out of the apartment and make the bed himself, then carefully wash and dry the breakfast dishes before setting out on the long crabwise uptown journey to Columbia.

Jeanne had no interest in his graduate studies. Her education, such as it was, had sunk in her without a trace; she could read and write and (though not easily) multiply and divide, but she never mentioned a book that she had liked or disliked and her knowledge of history embraced only such figures as Washington and Lincoln. Once, when Archer asked her to name the fifty states of the Union, with a bottle of Scotch for a prize if she could name them all, she was able to name only twenty-seven, and one of these turned out to be Omaha. Ross was often furious with her for being ignorant. "How can you stand knowing so little when you ought to know so much?" he would ask her, looking up from his reading. "I'd hate to have my mind as empty as yours is."

"You can be bright for both of us, baby."

Even his photography didn't interest her. He fashioned a makeshift darkroom out of a closet between the bedroom and bathroom and spent at least two hours of every day taking and developing pictures, and the most that she would say of the results was "That's very pretty," or "That's ugly. What do you see in such ugly things?" He took scores of pictures of her—a languorous odalisque, always fully clothed, for though she offered to pose for him in the nude, he rejected the offer with a taunt: "You're too fat."

"You never thought so before."

"You're not. Of course you're not. But I want your body to be mine. I don't want anyone to see it except me."

"Lots of people have seen it."

"Never any more."

"Then go back to taking pictures of chimneys and dead trees."

"What a bitchy thing to say. You don't care whether I become a good photographer or not."

She smiled and held out her arms. "Come to Mama."

Trembling with contempt and anger, he went to her.

The day of her death began like any other. She was, of course, behind schedule, and Ross shouted to her as she padded down the apartment-house stairs that he had a seminar that evening and wouldn't be back from Columbia until late. She stopped at the delicatessen and ordered a Danish and coffee ("Heavy on the cream"), which she savored slowly at her desk. Archer came in ahead of his usual time. The cutting down of the office staff had made him uneasy for Jeanne's sake, and he was determined that he and she should be seen to be getting a great deal of hard work accomplished. "I've already had my tea downstairs," he said.

"What a rotten liar you are."

"Listen, you know as well as I do what a panic my witless colleagues are in. They've lost two cents and they whimper like bankrupts."

"I'm not worrying. I'll go down and get us a special surprise. Something gooey."

"No, God damn it, you'll stay here and work." Archer's glasses slid to the very tip of his nose and hung there, and he was too distracted to push them back. "Please, Jeannie," said Foxy Grandpa, and because he had never said "please" and because he had never called her "Jeannie," she sat down beside him with pencil and paper and let him churn up the contents of his "in" and "out" baskets and fire off savage memos to his enemies until, to their astonishment, it was one o'clock.

"Watch the time," he said. "Be back by two."

"Time and tide wait for no man."

"I warn you, they'll throw you out."

"Let's cross that bridge when we come to it."

With a couple of girls from the office, she had lunch at Schrafft's, and perversely she took care to have her usual two vodka Martinis, followed by a glass of wine. When the other girls returned to the office, Jeanne drifted through midtown, window-shopping and enjoying the heat of the sun on her damp face and throat. She got back to the office to find an envelope waiting for her on the desk. It was her notice. Plainly, it had been prepared a day or two earlier, so plainly she had done well to dawdle over lunch. Coupled with her slight drunkenness, the sensation of having been fired—of having had something harsh and irrevocable happen—exhilarated her. She went into Archer's office to share this unexpected pleasure with him. "I feel—" she began, intending to tell him that she felt like a child let out of school, like a child at a circus, like a child with a red balloon, but seeing his face she guessed instantly what had befallen him, and in the same breath but in a different voice she ended, "Oh, Christ. I'm sorry."

No pipe, no glasses—why had he taken off his glasses? Had it been to keep them from being broken while they stripped him of his badge of office? He said, "They're making me put in for early retirement. I said I'd fight it, but of course I won't. I haven't anything to fight it with."

"Buy me a drink."

"You're already drunk. You ought to be ashamed."

"Now, Daddy-o."

"One drink, then, just to spit it in their eye."

In the little bar of his hotel, they sat drinking until after dark. Archer found his glasses in one pocket, his pipe in another. He never stopped talking, having thirty years of grievances to explore. He grew cheerful as he drank, and the worse the grievance the more uproarious it began to seem to them. Once or twice, he interrupted himself to say, "You don't have to stay and listen to all this dreary vomit, you know," and she smiled and patted his hand on the bar and, shaping the words with care, said, "Jeannie is a very, very, *very* good lis'ner." Around nine, they set out to find a place to eat. Holding tight to each other and tacking with brave abandon from one side of the pavement to the other, they made their way toward a restaurant that Jeanne remembered liking, a block or so from her apartment house. When they reached Jeanne's doorway without having located the restaurant, she suggested that he come up and let her cook supper for them. She worried a key out of her purse and between them they found the keyhole and unlocked the door. As they started up the stairs, Jeanne warned Archer that it would be a long climb and that he must stop talking in order to save his breath. The stairs proved even more treacherous than the sidewalk. Archer fell to his knees on almost every landing, when the counted-on next step failed to materialize. Occasionally, he took to his backside, bumping his way upward from tread to tread. Jeanne reached the fourth-floor landing ahead of him, and the door of the apartment was already open when, puffing with exertion, Archer arrived. He stumbled past Jeanne into the living room. "Welcome!" he said to her as she followed him in, and then, "Bathroom?"

Leaving the bathroom, Archer took a wrong turn, wheeled into the dark bedroom, tripped over a camera tripod, and crashed to the floor, carrying the tripod and a small table with him. Jeanne hurried to him from the kitchen, switching on lights as she went. Archer was moaning and Jeanne was laughing as she gathered him up off the floor and propped him, a crumpled tweed sack, on the edge of the bed. She peeled off his jacket, trousers, and shoes, and pushed and rolled him onto the far side of the bed. "Take forty winks while I get supper," she said. Archer made no answer. Curled with his face to the wall and holding his boney, bruised knees in his hands, he was already asleep.

Jeanne went to the bathroom to sprinkle cold water on her face. She felt very drunk and very cheerful and only a little sick as yet. Rocking from foot to foot, she stared at her bathrobe hanging in its accustomed place on a hook on the back of the bathroom door. Even sober, she had room in her mind for but one thought at a time; the bathrobe before her, she no longer remembered her plan for making supper. She washed her hands and brushed her teeth, fumblingly undressed herself, and returned to the bedroom. With a sigh of pleasure, she lay down naked upon the bed and crooked her arm over her eyes to ward off the light. As she fell asleep, she turned on her side and drew up against the soft warmth of her breasts Archer's wiry little body. And there they lay when Ross came back at midnight and walked into the apartment ablaze with lights and called her name.

OBESITY AND EATING

*Internal and external cues differentially affect the
eating behavior of obese and normal subjects.*

by Stanley Schachter

Current conceptions of hunger control mechanisms indicate that food deprivation leads to various peripheral
physiological changes such as modification of blood con-
stituents, increase in gastric motility, changes in body tem-
perature, and the like. By means of some still debated
mechanism, these changes are detected by a hypothalamic
feeding center. Presumably some or all facets of this activated machinery lead the organism to search out and consume food. There appears to be no doubt that peripheral
physiological changes and activation of the hypothalamic
feeding center are inevitable consequences of food deprivation. On the basis of current knowledge, however, one
may ask, when this biological machinery is activated, do we
necessarily describe ourselves as hungry, and eat? For most
of us raised on the notion that hunger is the most primitive
of motives, wired into the animal and unmistakable in its
cues, the question may seem far-fetched, but there is increasing reason to suspect that there are major individual
differences in the extent to which these physiological
changes are associated with the desire to eat.

On the clinical level, the analyst Hilde Bruch *(1)* has
observed that her obese patients literally do not know when
they are physiologically hungry. To account for this obser-
vation she suggests that, during childhood, these patients
were not taught to discriminate between hunger and such
states as fear, anger, and anxiety. If this is so, these people
may be labeling almost any state of arousal "hunger," or,
alternatively, labeling no internal state "hunger."

If Bruch's speculations are correct, it should be anticipated that the set of physiological symptoms which are considered characteristic of food deprivation are not labeled "hunger" by the obese. In other words the obese literally may not know when they are physiologically hungry. For at least one of the presumed physiological correlates of food deprivation, this does appear to be the case. In an absorbing study, Stunkard *(2, 3)* has related gastric motility to self-reports of hunger in 37 obese subjects and 37 subjects of normal size. A subject, who had eaten no breakfast, came to the laboratory at 9 A.M.; he swallowed a gastric balloon, and for 4 hours Stunkard continuously recorded gastric motility. Every 15 minutes the subject was asked if he was hungry. He answered "yes" or "no," and that is all there was to the study. We have, then, a record of the extent to which a subject's self-report of hunger corresponds to his gastric motility. The results show (i) that obese and normal subjects do not differ significantly in degree of gastric motility, and (ii) that, when the stomach is not contracting, the reports of obese and normal subjects are quite similar, both groups reporting hunger roughly 38 percent of the time. When the stomach is contracting, however, the reports of the two groups differ markedly. For normal subjects, self-report of hunger coincides with gastric motility 71 percent of the time. For the obese, the percentage is only 47.6. Stunkard's work seems to indicate that obese and normal subjects do not refer to the same bodily state when they use the term *hunger.*

Effects of Food Deprivation and Fear

If this inference is correct, we should anticipate that, if we were to directly manipulate gastric motility and the other symptoms that we associate with hunger, we would, for normal subjects, be directly manipulating feelings of hunger and eating behavior. For the obese there would be no correspondence between manipulated internal state and eating behavior. To test these expectations, Goldman, Gordon, and I *(4)* performed an experiment in which bodily state was manipulated by two means—(i) by the obvious technique of manipulating food deprivation, so that some subjects had empty stomachs and others had full stomachs before eating; (ii) by manipulating fear, so that some subjects were badly frightened and others were quite calm immediately before eating. Carlson *(5)* has indicated that fear inhibits gastric motility; Cannon *(6)* also has demonstrated that fear inhibits motility, and has shown that it leads to the liberation, from the liver, of sugar into the blood. Hypoglycemia and gastric contractions are generally considered the chief peripheral physiological correlates of food deprivation.

Our experiment was conducted under the guise of a study of taste. A subject came to the laboratory in mid afternoon or evening. He had been called the previous evening and asked not to eat the meal (lunch or dinner) preceding his appointment at the laboratory. The experiment was introduced as a study of "the interdependence of the basic human senses—of the way in which the stimulation of one sense affects another." Specifically, the subject was told that this study would be concerned with "the effects of tactile stimulation on the way things taste."

It was explained that all subjects had been asked not to eat a meal before coming to the laboratory because "in any scientific experiment it is necessary that the subjects be as similar as possible in all relevant ways. As you probably know from your own experience," the experimenter continued, "an important factor in determining how things taste is what you have recently eaten." The introduction over, the experimenter then proceeded as follows.

For the "full stomach" condition he said to the subject, "In order to guarantee that your recent taste experiences are similar to those of other subjects who have taken part in this experiment, we should now like you to eat exactly the same thing they did. Just help yourself to the roast beef sandwiches on the table. Eat as much as you want—till you're full."

For the "empty stomach" condition, the subjects, of course, were not fed.

Next, the subject was seated in front of five bowls of crackers and told, "We want you to taste five different kinds of crackers and tell us how they taste to you." The experimenter then gave the subject a long set of rating scales and said, "We want you to judge each cracker on the dimensions (salty, cheesy, garlicky, and so on) listed on this sheet. Taste as many or as few of the crackers of each type as you want in making your judgments; the important thing is that your ratings be as accurate as possible."

Before permitting the subject to eat, the experimenter continued with the next stage of the experiment—the manipulation of fear.

"As I mentioned," he said, "our primary interest in this experiment is the effect of tactile stimulation on taste. Electric stimulation is the means we use to excite your skin receptors. We use this method in order to carefully control the amount of stimulation you receive."

For the "low fear" condition the subject was told, "For the effects in which we are interested, we need to use only the lowest level of stimulation. At most you will feel a slight tingle. Probably you will feel nothing at all. We are only interested in the effect of very weak stimulation."

For the "high fear" condition the experimenter pointed to a large black console loaded with electrical junk and said, "That machine is the one we will be using. I am afraid that these shocks will be painful. For them to have any effect on your taste sensations, the voltage must be rather high. There will, of course, be no permanent damage. Do you have a heart condition?" A large electrode connected to the console was then attached to each of the subject's ankles, and the experimenter concluded, "The best way for us to test the effect of tactile stimulation is to have you rate the crackers now, before the electric shock, and then rate them again, after the shock, to see what changes in your ratings the shock has made."

The subject then proceeded to taste and rate crackers for 15 minutes, under the impression that this was a taste test; meanwhile we were simply counting the number of crackers he ate *(7)*. We then had measures of the amounts eaten by subjects who initially had either empty or full stomachs and who were initially either frightened or calm. There were of course, two types of subjects; obese subjects (from 14 percent to 75 percent overweight) and normal subject (from 8 percent underweight to 9 percent overweight).

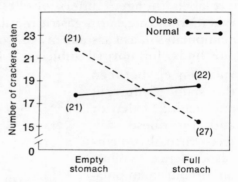

Fig. 1. Effects of preliminary eating on the amounts eaten during the experiment by normal and obese subjects. Numbers in parentheses are numbers of subjects.

To review expectations: If we were correct in thinkng that the obese do not label as hunger the bodily states associated with food deprivation, then our several experimental manipulations should have had no effects on the amount eaten by obese subjects; on the other hand, the eating behavior of normal subjects should have directly paralleled the effects of the manipulations on bodily state.

It will be a surprise to no one to learn, from Fig. 1, that the normal subjects ate considerably fewer crackers when their stomachs were full than when their stomachs were empty. The results for obese subjects stand in fascinating contrast. They ate as much—in fact, slightly more—when their stomachs were full as when they were empty (interaction $P < .05$). Obviously the actual state of the stomach has nothing to do with the eating behavior of the obese.

In Fig. 2, pertaining to the effect of fear, we note an

analogous picture. Fear markedly decreased the number of crackers the normal subjects ate but had no effect on the number eaten by the obese (interaction $P < .01$). Again, there was a small, though nonsignificant, reversal: the fearful obese ate slightly more than the calm obese.

It seems clear that the set of bodily symptoms the subject labels "hunger" differs for obese and normal subjects. Whether one measures gastric motility, as Stunkard did, or manipulates it, as I assume my co-workers and I have done, one finds, for normal subjects, a high degree of correspondence between the state of the gut and eating behavior and, for obese subjects, virtually no correspondence. While all of our manipulations have had a major effect on the amounts eaten by normal subjects, nothing that we have done has had a substantial effect on the amounts eaten by obese subjects.

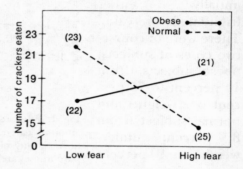

Fig. 2. Effects of fear on the amounts eaten by normal and obese subjects. Numbers in parentheses are numbers of subjects.

Effects of the Circumstances of Eating

With these facts in mind, let us turn to the work of Hashim and Van Itallie *(8)* of the Nutrition Clinic, St. Luke's Hospital, New York City. Their findings may be summarized as follows: virtually everything these workers do seems to have a major effect on the eating behavior of the obese and almost no effect on the eating behavior of the normal subject.

These researchers have prepared a bland liquid diet similar to commercial preparations such as vanilla-flavored Nutrament or Metrecal. The subjects are restricted to this monotonous diet for periods ranging from a week to several months. They can eat as much or as little of it as they want. Some of the subjects get a pitcher full and pour themselves a meal any time they wish. Other subjects are fed by a machine which delivers a mouthful every time the subject presses a button. With either feeding technique, the eating situation has the following characteristics. (i) The food itself is unappealing. (ii) Eating is entirely self-determined: whether or not the subject eats, how much he eats, and when he eats are matters decided by him and no one else. Absolutely no pressure is brought to bear to limit his consumption. (iii) The eating situation is devoid of any social or domestic trappings. It is basic eating; it will keep the subject alive, but it's not much fun.

To date, six grossly obese and five normal individuals have been subjects in these studies. In Fig. 3 the eating curves for a typical pair of subjects over a 21-day period are plotted. Both subjects were healthy people who lived in the hospital during the entire study. The obese subject was a 52-year-old woman, 5 feet 3 inches (1.6 meters) tall, who weighed 307 pounds (138 kilograms) on admission. The normal subject was a 30-year-old male, 5 feet 7 inches tall, who weighed 132 pounds.

The subject's estimated daily caloric intake before entering the hospital (as determined from a detailed interview) is plotted at the left in Fig. 3. Each subject, while in the hospital but before entering upon the experimental regime, was fed a general hospital diet. The obese subject was placed on a 2400-calorie diet for 7 days and a 1200-calorie diet for the next 8 days. As may be seen in Fig. 3, she ate everything on her tray throughout this 15 day period. The normal subject was placed on a 2400-calorie diet for 2 days, and he too ate everything.

With the beginning of the experiment proper, the difference in the eating behavior of the two subjects was dramatic and startling. The food consumption of the obese subject dropped precipitately the moment she entered upon the experimental regime, and it remained at an incredibly low level for the duration of the experiment. This effect is so dramatic that the weight of one obese subject who took part in the experiment for 8 months dropped from 410 to 190 pounds. On the other hand, the food consumption of the normal subject of Fig. 3 dropped slightly on the first 2 days, then returned to a fairly steady 2300 grams or so of food a day. The curves for these two subjects are typical. Each of the six obese subjects has manifested this marked and persistent decrease in food consumption during the experiment; each of the normal subjects has steadily consumed about his normal amount of food.

Before suggesting possible interpretations, I should note certain marked differences between these two groups of subjects. Most important, the obese subjects had come to the clinic for help in solving their weight problem and were, of course, motivated to lose weight. The normal subjects were simple volunteers. Doubtless this difference could account for the observed difference in eating behavior during the experiment,

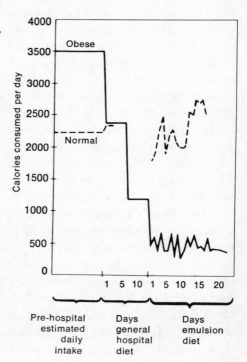

Fig. 3. The effects of an emulsion diet on the amounts eaten by an obese and a normal subject.

and until obese volunteers, unconcerned with their weight, are used as subjects in similar studies, we cannot be sure of the interpretation of this phenomenon. However, I think we should not, solely on grounds of methodological fastidiousness, dismiss these findings. It was concern with weight that brought these obese subjects to the clinic. Each of them, before entering the hospital and while in the hospital before being put on the experimental diet, was motivated to lose weight. Yet, despite this motivation, none of these subjects had been capable of restricting his diet at home, and each of them, when fed the general hospital diet, had eaten everything on his tray. Only when the food was dull and the act of eating was self-initiated and devoid of any ritual trappings did the obese subject, motivated or not, severely limit his consumption.

Internal and External Control

On the one hand, then, our experiments indicate virtually no relationship between internal physiological state and the eating behavior of the obese subject; on the other hand, these case studies seem to indicate a close tie between the eating behavior of the obese and what might be called the circumstances of eating. When the food is dull and the eating situation is uninteresting, the obese subject eats virtually nothing. For the normal subject, the situation is just the reverse: his eating behavior seems directly linked to his physiological state but is relatively unaffected by the external circumstances or the ritual associated with eating.

Given this set of facts it seems clear that eating is triggered by different sets of stimuli in obese and normal subjects. Indeed, there is growing reason to suspect that the eating behavior of the obese is relatively unrelated to any internal state but is, in large part, under external control, being initiated and terminated by stimuli external to the organism. Let me give a few examples. A person whose eating behavior is under external control will stroll by a pastry shop, find the food in the window irresistible, and, even if he has recently eaten, go in and buy something. He will pass by a hamburger stand, smell the broiling meat, and, even though he has just eaten, buy a hamburger. Obviously such external factors—smell, sight, taste, other people's actions—to some extent affect anyone's eating. However, in normal individuals such external factors interact with internal state. They may affect what, where, and how much the normal individual eats, but they do so chiefly when he is in a state of physiological hunger. For the obese, I suggest, internal state is irrelevant and eating is determined largely by external factors.

This hypothesis obviously fits the data presented here, as well it should, since it is an *ad hoc* construction designed specifically to fit these data. Let us see, then, what independent support there is for the hypothesis, and where the hypothesis leads.

Effects of Manipulating Time

Among the multitude of external food-relevant cues, one of the most intriguing is the passage of time. Everyone "knows" that 4 to 6 hours after eating his last meal he should eat his next one. Everyone "knows" that, within narrow limits, there are set times for eating regular meals. We should, then, expect that if we manipulate time we should be able to manipulate the eating behavior of the obese subjects. In order to do this, Gross and I *(a)* simply gimmicked two clocks so that one ran at half normal speed and the other, at twice normal speed. A subject arrives at 5:00 p.m., ostensibly to take part in an experiment on the relationship of base levels of autonomic reactivity to personality factors. He is ushered into a windowless room containing nothing but electronic equipment and a clock. Electrodes are put on his wrists, his watch is removed "so that it will not get gummed up with electrode jelly," and he is connected to a polygraph. All this takes 5 minutes, and at 5:05 he is left alone, with nothing to do for a true

30 minutes, while ostensibly we are getting a record of galvanic skin response and cardiac rate in a subject at rest. There are two experimental conditions. In one, the experimenter returns after a true 30 minutes and the clock reads 5:20. In the other, the clock reads 6:05, which is normal dinner time for most subjects. In both cases the experimenter is carrying a box of crackers and nibbling a cracker as he comes into the room; he puts the box down, invites the subject to help himself, removes the electrodes from the subject's wrists, and proceeds with personality testing for exactly 5 minutes. This done, he gives the subject a personality inventory which he is to complete and leaves him alone with the box of crackers for another true 10 minutes. There are two groups of subjects—normal and obese—and the only datum we collect is the weight of the box of crackers before and after the subject has had a chance at it.

If these ideas on internal and external controls of eating behavior are correct, normal subjects, whose eating behavior is presumably linked to internal state, should be relatively unaffected by the manipulation and should eat roughly the same number of crackers regardless of whether the clock reads 5:20 or 6:05. The obese, on the other hand, whose eating behavior is presumably under external control, should eat very few crackers when the clock reads 5:20 and a great many crackers when it reads 6:05.

The data of Fig. 4 do indeed indicate that the obese subjects eat almost twice as many crackers when they think the time is 6:05 as they do when they believe it to be 5:20. For normal subjects, the trend is just the reverse (interaction = .002)—an unanticipated finding but one which seems embarrassingly simple to explain, as witness the several normal subjects who thought the time was 6:05 and politely refused the crackers, saying, "No thanks, I don't want to spoil my dinner." Obviously cognitive factors affected the eating behavior of both the normal and the obese subjects, but there was a vast difference. While the manipulation of the clock served to trigger or stimulate eating among the obese, it had the opposite effect on normal subjects, most of whom at this hour were, we presume, physiologically hungry, aware that they would eat dinner very shortly, and unwilling to spoil their dinner by filling up on crackers.

Effects of Taste

In another study, Nisbett *(10)* examined the effects of taste on eating behavior. Nisbett reasoned that taste, like the sight or smell of food, is essentially an external stimulus to eating. Nisbett, in his experiment, also extended the range of weight deviation by including a group of underweight subjects as well as obese and normal subjects. His purpose in so doing was to examine the hypothesis that the relative potency of external versus internal controls is a dimension directly related to the degree of overweight. If the hypothesis was correct, he reasoned, the taste of food would have the greatest impact on the amounts eaten by obese subjects and the least impact on the amounts eaten by underweight subjects. To test this, Nisbett had his subjects eat as much as they wanted of one of two kinds of vanilla ice cream; one was a delicious and expensive product, the other an acrid concoction of cheap vanilla and quinine which he called "vanilla bitters." The effects of taste are presented in Fig. 5, in which the subjects' ratings of how good or bad the ice cream is are plotted against the amount eaten. As may be seen in Fig. 5, when the ice cream was rated "fairly good" or better, the obese subjects ate considerably more than the normal subjects did; these, in turn, ate more than the underweight subjects did. When the ice cream was rated "not very good" or worse, the ordering tended to reverse: the underweight subjects ate more than either the normal or the obese subjects. This experiment, then, indicates that the external, or at least nonvisceral, cue *taste* does have differential effects on the eating behavior of underweight, normal, and obese subjects.

The indications, from Nisbett's experiment, that the degree of dependence on external cues relative to internal cues varies with deviation from normal weight are intriguing, for, if further work supports this hypothesis, we may have the beginnings of a plausible explanation of why the thin are thin and the fat are fat. We know from Carlson's work *(5)* that gastric contractions cease after a small amount of food has been introduced into the stomach. To the extent that such contractions are directly related to the hunger "experience"—to the extent that a person's eating is under internal control—he should "eat like a bird," eating only enough to stop the contractions. Eating beyond this point should be a function of external cues—the taste, sight, and smell of food. Individuals whose eating is externally controlled, then, should find it hard to stop eating. This hypothesis may account for the notorious "binge" eating of the obese *(11)* or the monumental meals described in loving detail by students *(12)* of the great, fat gastronomic magnificoes.

This rough attempt to explain why the obese are obese in itself raises intriguing questions. For example, does the external control of eating behavior inevitably lead to obesity? It is evident, I believe, that not only is such a linkage logically not inevitable but that the condition of external control of eating may in rare but specifiable circumstances lead to emaciation. A person whose eating is externally controlled should eat and grow fat when food-related cues are abundant and when he is fully aware of them. However, when such cues are lacking or when for some reason, such as withdrawal or depression, the individual is unaware of the cues, the person under external control would, one would expect, not eat, and, if the condition persisted, would grow "concentration-camp" thin. From study of the clinical literature one does get the impression that there is an odd but distinct relationship between obesity and extreme emaciation. For example, 11 of 21 subjects of case studies discussed by Bliss and Branch in *Anorexia Nervosa*

(13) were, at some time in their lives, obese. In the case of eight of these 11 subjects, anorexia was preceded and accompanied by either marked withdrawal or intense depression. In contrast, intense attacks of anxiety or nervousness [states which our experiment *(4)* suggests would inhibit eating in normal individuals] seem to be associated with the development of anorexia among most of the ten subjects who were originally of normal size.

At this point, these speculations are simply idea-spinning—fun, but ephemeral. Let us return to the results of the studies described so far. These can be quickly summarized as follows.

1) Physiological correlates of food deprivation, such as gastric motility, are directly related to eating behavior and to the reported experience of hunger in normal subjects but unrelated in obese subjects *(3, 4)*.

2) External or nonvisceral cues, such as smell, taste, the sight of other people eating, and the passage of time, affect eating behavior to a greater extent in obese subjects than in normal subjects *(8-10)*.

Obesity and Fasting

Given these basic facts, their implications have ramifications in almost any area pertaining to food and eating, and some of our studies have been concerned with the implications of these experimental results for eating behavior on a variety of nonlaboratory settings. Thus, Goldman, Jaffa, and I *(14)* have studied fasting on Yom Kippur, the Jewish Day of Atonement, on which the orthodox Jew is supposed to go without food for 24 hours. Reasoning that, on this occasion, food-relevant external cues are particularly scarce, one would expect obese Jews to be more likely to fast than normal Jews. In a study of 296 religious Jewish college students (defined as Jewish college students who had been to a synagogue at least once during the preceding year on occasions other than a wedding or a bar mitzvah), this proves to be the case, for 83.3 percent of obese Jews fasted, as compared with 68.8 percent of normal Jews (*P* < .05).

Further, this external-internal control schema leads to the prediction that fat, fasting Jews who spend a great deal of time in the synagogue on Yom Kippur will suffer less from fasting than fat, fasting Jews who spend little time in the synagogue. There should be no such relationship for normal fasting Jews. Obviously, there will be far fewer food-related cues in the synagogue than on the street or at home. Therefore, for obese Jews, the likelihood that the impulse to eat will be triggered is greater outside of the synagogue than within it. For normal Jews, this distinction is of less importance. In or out of the synagogue, stomach pangs are stomach pangs. Again, the data support the expectation. When the number of hours in the synagogue is correlated with self-ratings of the unpleasantness of fasting, for obese subjects the correlation is −.50, whereas for normal subjects the correlation is only −.18. In a test of the difference between correlations, *P* = .03. Obviously, for the obese, the more time the individual spends in the synagogue, the less of an ordeal fasting is. For normals, the number of hours in the synagogue has little to do with the difficulty of the fast.

Obesity and Choice of Eating Place

In another study *(14)* we examined the relationship of obesity to choice of eating places. From Nisbett's findings on taste, it seemed a plausible guess that the obese would be more drawn to good restaurants and more repelled by bad ones than normal subjects would be. At Columbia, students have the option of eating in the university dining halls or in any of the many restaurants that surround the campus. At Columbia, as probably at every similar institution in the United States, students have a low opinion of the institution's food. If a freshman elects to eat in a dormitory dining hall, he may, if he chooses, join a prepayment food plan at the beginning of the school year. Any time after 1 November he may, by paying a penalty of $15, cancel his food contract. If we accept prevailing campus opinion of the institution's food as being at all realistically based, we should anticipate that those for whom taste or food quality is most important will be the most likely to let their food contracts expire. Obese freshmen, then, should be more likely to drop out of the food plan than normal

freshmen. Again, the data support the expectation: 86.5 percent of fat freshman cancel their contracts as compared with 67.1 percent of normal freshmen ($P > .05$). Obesity does to some extent serve as a basis for predicting who will choose to eat institutional food.

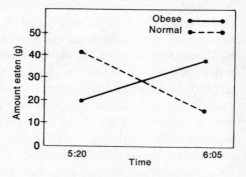

Fig. 4. The effects of manipulation of time on the amounts eaten by obese and normal subjects.

Obesity and Adjustment to New Eating Schedules

In the final study in this series *(14)* we examined the relationship of obesity to the difficulty of adjusting to new eating schedules imposed by time-zone changes. This study involved an analysis of data collected by the medical department of Air France in a study of physiological effects of time-zone changes on 236 flight personnel assigned to the Paris–New York and Paris–Montreal flights. Most of these flights leave Paris around noon, French time; fly for approximately 8 hours; and land in North America sometime between 2:00 and 3:00 p.m. Eastern time. Flight-crew members eat lunch shortly after takeoff and, being occupied with landing preparations, are not served another meal during the flight. They land some 7 hours after their last meal, at a time that is later than the local lunch hour and earlier than the local dinner time.

Though this study was not directly concerned with eating behavior, the interviewers systematically noted all individuals who volunteered the information that they "suffered from the discordance between their physiological state and meal time in America" *(15)*. One would anticipate that the fatter individuals, being sensitive to external cues (local meal hours) rather than internal ones, would adapt most readily to local eating schedules and be least likely to complain of the discrepancy between American meal times and physiological state.

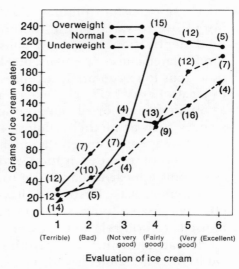

Fig. 5. The effects of food quality on the amounts eaten by obese, normal, and underweight subjects. Numbers in parentheses are numbers of subjects.

Given the physical requirements involved in the selection of aircrews, there are, of course, relatively few really obese people in this sample. However, the results of Nisbett's experiment *(10)* indicate that the degree of reliance on external relative to internal cues may well be a dimension which varies with the degrees of deviation from normal weight. It seems reasonable, then, to anticipate that, even within a restricted sample, there will be differences in response between the heavier and the lighter members of the sample. This is the case. In comparing the 101 flight personnel who are overweight (0.1 to 29 percent overweight) with the 135 who are not overweight (0 to 25 percent underweight), we find that 11.9 percent of the overweight complain as compared with 25.3 percent of the nonoverweight ($P <$ .01). It does appear that the fatter were less troubled by the effects of time changes on eating than the thinner flyers (16).

These persistent findings that the obese are relatively insensitive to variations in the physiological correlates of food deprivation but highly sensitive to environmental, food-related cues is, perhaps, one key to understanding the notorious long-run ineffectiveness of virtually all attempts to treat obesity (17). The use of anorexigenic drugs such as amphetamine or of bulk-producing, nonnutritive substances such as methyl cellulose is based on the premise that such agents dampen the intensity of the physiological symptoms of food deprivation. Probably they do, but these symptoms appear to have little to do with whether or not a fat person eats. Restricted, low-calorie diets should be effective just so long as the obese dieter is able to blind himself to food-relevant cues or so long as he exists in a world barren of such cues. In the Hashim and Van Itallie study (8), the subjects did, in fact, live in such a world. Restricted to a Metrecal-like diet and to a small hospital ward, all the obese subjects lost impressive amounts of weight. However, on their return to normal living, to a man they returned to their original weights.

References and Notes

1. H. Bruch, *Psychiat. Quart.* **35,** 458 (1961).
2. A. Stunkard, *Psychosomat. Med.* **21,** 281 (1959).
3. —— and C. Koch, *Arch. Genet. Psychiat.* **11,** 74 (1964).
4. S. Schachter, R. Goldman, A. Gordon, *J. Personality Soc. Psychol.,* in press.
5. A. J. Carlson, *Control of Hunger in Health and Disease* (Univ. of Chicago Press, Chicago, 1916).
6. W. B. Cannon, *Bodily Changes in Pain, Hunger, Fear and Rage* (Appleton, New York, 1915).

7. It is a common belief among researchers in the field of obesity that the sensitivity of their fat subjects makes it impossible to study their eating behavior experimentally—hence this roundabout way of measuring eating; the subjects in this study are taking a "taste test," not "eating."

8. S. A. Hashim and T. B. Van Itallie, *Ann. N. Y. Acad. Sci.* **131,** 654 (1965).

9. S. Schachter and L. Gross, *J. Personality Soc. Psychol.,* in press.

10. R. E. Nisbett, *ibid.,* in press.

11. A. Stunkard, *Amer. J. Psychiat.* **118,** 212 (1961).

12. L. Beebe, *The Big Spenders* (Doubleday, New York, 1966).

13. E. L. Bliss and C. H. Branch, *Anorexia Nervosa* (Hoeber, New York, 1960).

14. R. Goldman, M. Jaffa, S. Schachter. *J. Personality Soc. Psychol.,* in press.

15. J. Lavernhe and E. Lafontaine (Air France), personal communication.

16. Obviously, I do not mean to imply that the *only* explanation of the results of these three nonlaboratory studies lies in this formulation of the external-internal control of eating behavior. These studies were deliberately designed to test implications of this general schema in field settings. As with any field research, alternative explanations of the findings are legion, and, within the context of any specific study, impossible to rule out. Alternative formulations of this entire series of studies are considered in the original papers [see Schachter *et al. (4* and *9),* Nisbett *(10),* and Goldman *et al. (14)*].

17. A.Stunkard and M. McLaren-Hume, *Arch. Internal Med.* **103,** 79 (1959); A. R. Feinstein, *J. Chronic Diseases* **11,** 349 (1960).

18. Much of the research described in this article was supported by grants G23758 and GS732 from the National Science Foundation.

THIN FAT PEOPLE

from EATING DISORDERS: Obesity, Anorexia
Nervosa and the Person Within

by **Hilde Bruch**

Saul Bellow's brief sketch of Angela, Mr. Sammler's niece, could easily be applied to countless American women. Her appearance and behavior sound familiar to us, though it impressed her uncle as strange (1).

> Angela was in her thirties now, independently wealthy, with ruddy skin, gold-whitish hair, big lips. She was afraid of obesity. She either fasted or ate like a stevedore. She trained in a fashionable gym. She wore the odd stylish things which Sammler noted with detached and purified dryness, as if from a different part of the universe. What were those, white-kid buskins? What were those tights—sheer, opaque? Where did they lead? That effect of the hair called frosting, that color under the lioness's muzzle, that swagger to enhance the natural power of the bust! Her plastic coat inspired by cubists or Mondrians, geometrical black and white forms; her trousers by Courrèges and Pucci.

In spite of her up-to-date, mod appearance and well-controlled figure, Angela was not happy. She was always getting involved in wild schemes to improve herself and the world, and she found solace in going to a psychiatrist. This, too, has a familiar ring. My own knowledge about the seemingly successful but desperate fight against obesity comes from many patients who came for psychiatric treatment for a variety of reasons, and who on first contact did not seem to be concerned with their weight at all.

Fat people are apt to blame all their difficulties on being fat and they hope for a new lease on life after they get thin. Many begin reducing confident of finding the pot of gold

190

at the end of the rainbow. Few reach the goal; otherwise we would not be so concerned about fat people's inability to stick to a diet. But there are some who follow through, who can deny their desire for food and achieve the beautiful slim figure that is supposed to be the magic key to the doorway to success and happiness. And it may be that there are many for whom things work out this way; it so happens that I am not familiar with this course of events. People who are successful and stay reduced and are relaxed about it do not go to physicians with their weight problems; they certainly will not come to a psychiatrist.

From my observations there are three outcomes for people who reduce with the unrealistic goal of expecting a changed life before they have experienced the inner emotional changes which make these new adjustments possible. The great majority will try and try, will lose some weight and then, suddenly they will give up and regain and often overshoot their former weight. For others the stress of starving themselves, the loss of their size, the new real or imagined expectations may prove too much, and serious emotional disturbances, even frank psychotic behavior, may break through.

There is a third group of people who succeed in becoming and staying thin, but whose conflicts are far from solved by having lost weight. On the contrary, their difficulties now have a chance to flourish, since the ugliness of being fat no longer prevents them from putting their unrealistic dreams to the test. Such people, though they no longer look obese, are far from cured; they still resemble fat people with all their unsolved problems, conflicts, and exaggerated expectations. Only they no longer *show* their fat. It is to this group that I wish to apply the term *Thin Fat People,* an expression I borrowed from Heckel, who stated in 1911 that we cannot consider a fat person cured, even though he has lost his weight, unless all the other functional symptoms have also disappeared (3). Loss of weight alone represents a pseudo-cure. The patient becomes "un obèse amaigri; mais il est toujours un obèse." The charac-

teristics of a good cure, Heckel says, are that it should be
lasting and that it should not make unreasonable demands
on the patient.

Sometimes being slim is a professional necessity. I know
a most attractive young girl who had made a place for
herself as a model. She is pretty in a petite way, but by any
standard of medical appraisal she is definitely undernour-
ished, as is Twiggy, the most famous of the starved models.
However, now that she is 19, it is doubtful whether she will
be able to continue her career; whenever she applies for
a job she is looked over and told that she must watch her
figure, that she is getting too fat. She considers the great
hazard of her profession the strain of constant fatigue.
Only after we had discussed the details of her fatigue did
she realize that most of it was due to being hungry all the
time. She had observed that other young girls working as
models frequently would faint and she was alarmed when
she fainted for the first time, but then recognized it for what
it was. In view of her enjoyment of the job, the good pay,
and the sense of accomplishment she derived from being
independent from her family she feels it worth the price,
at least for a few more years.

A young woman with a magnificent voice noted a tumor,
which turned out to be malignant, at exactly the time when
she was first recognized nationwide as an artist. After the
operation, she continued her career and achieved stardom,
but was unhappy about her increasing weight. Though she
"knew" better, she acted under the inner conviction that
she *had* to eat to maintain her health, so that she would not
suffer a recurrence. Once she felt "safe," more than five
years after the operation, she decided to lose weight and
consulted an experienced physician who supported her
during an episode of resolute dieting. She brought her
weight down to ten pounds below her former weight and
has maintained it at this low level for several years. She
enjoys her youthful, slim figure and feels that all the personal and professional satisfaction she gains from it is well

worth the sacrifice of being continuously food and weight conscious.

A friend of mine, psychologically gifted and probably more perceptive than most people, spoke about her own efforts to keep her weight under control, and what it meant to lose the extra ten pounds that accumulated during a winter of sedentary habits and party-going. "I don't mind cutting out sweets or any one particular item. What I resent about dieting is that it makes one so terribly self-centered, so much aware of oneself and one's body, so preoccupied with things that apply to oneself only that there is scarcely any energy left to be really spontaneous, relaxed, and outgoing. It starts with thinking about what to eat and what not to eat, and gradually goes over to other fields, and it is this aspect that makes me resent dieting; it makes me less of a human being.

"Of course I don't want to look sloppy and fat and I want my husband and children to enjoy going out with me—but I sometimes wonder whether it is worth the strain and effort and whether I have the right to pay so much attention to my appearance at the price of being an unresponsive mother."

This woman had no tendency to obesity. The extra weight was not noticeable unless she drew attention to it. Her desire to stay slim and not to look dowdy is also that of a well-adjusted person, not of the fashion-plate compulsive type who wants to be thin for thinness's sake, as a matter of thoughtless conformity. But even for such a woman, pushing her weight below the level that is really comfortable for her involves a noticeable mental strain.

Problems become more severe for those who have a tendency to be obese, or who use overeating to ameliorate serious emotional tension. I am most familiar with this pseudo-thinness from my contact with the relatives of fat young people. Whenever one hears a thin, even scrawny-looking mother speak with particular vehemence and disgust about the fatness of her child it is not a far-fetched guess (and one easily confirmed) that this mother owes her fashionable figure to eternal vigilance and conscientious, semistarvation dieting. Fathers are not exempt from this rule. It seems to me that the hostile emotional overcharge is related to envy in the parent about the child's daring to satisfy his appetite and impulses. The parents' rage reveals their shame that the child's fatness exposes the despised family endowment. It is in families with this intense hostility about obesity that I have most often seen a malignant development of childhood obesity, with schizophrenic or anorexia nervosa as the final outcome.

Mrs. Jones is an example of such a mother. She is pretty and slim and considers it an insult and a disgrace for the whole family that her twelve-year-old daughter is fat, moody, and unpopular. At first there was nothing to indicate that the mother herself has a weight problem—her weight has been stable for many years at 110 pounds. The first inkling of something wrong was the fact that all the complaints about her daughter's lack of attention and carelessness had to do with food. For example, one day while she was at the hairdresser's she sent her daughter to a certain delicatessen store for a sandwich, and the girl came back with a sandwich from another store which was not up to the mother's expectations. She made a terrible scene, shouting: "Do you expect me to eat *dirt?*" She takes pride in being so particular about food and will return a dish in a restaurant that is not absolutely perfect, though her husband and friends find her behavior embarrassing. Gradually she revealed that she had been quite plump before her marriage, that she had slimmed down for the wedding and has watched every bite she eats ever since. She is extraordinarily preoccupied with food, and has replaced the quantity she has sacrificed by the demand for superfine quality.

She is overly perfectionistic in her whole approach to her daughter, who complains: "Yes, I know, you love me a lot—you love me so much that you expect me to be perfect." In every respect this mother had tried to be perfect in her role, raising her child by the book, "Whatever was fashionable at that time." She was aware that her need to satisfy her own mother conflicted with her modern views and created confusion for the child. She felt her mother was lonely and unhappy, therefore she permitted her to overindulge the little girl, though the grandmother handled her quite differently from the mother. The girl was overly attached to the grandmother and reacted with real depression to her death. It was following this loss, when she was five years old, that the girl grew fat and became moody and withdrawn, and this provoked the mother's campaign to demand perfection.

Many women make a fetish of being thin and follow reducing diets without awareness of or regard for the fact that they can do so only at the price of continuous strain and tension and some degree of ill health. There are millions of young girls and women who starve themselves in order to look like these envied models for whom slimness is a well-paid professional pose. Ordinary young women do not get paid for being slim. When they become young mothers they will complain continuously about fatigue, about their children's problems, and about their own irritability. Little attention has been paid to the fact that their attempt to fulfill fashion's demands to be skinny is directly related to these problems. Having grown up with the concept that thinness is identical with beauty and attractiveness and is desirable for its own sake, they have become used to living on a semistarvation diet, never eating more than their bony figures show. Never having permitted themselves to eat adequately, they are unaware of how much of their tension, bad disposition, irritability, and inability to pursue an educational or professional goal is the direct result of chronic undernutrition.

It is impossible to assess the cost in serenity, relaxation, and efficiency of this abnormal, overslim, fashionable appearance. It produces serious psychological tensions to feel compelled to be thinner than one's natural make-up and style of living demand. There is a great deal of talk about the weakness and self-indulgence of overweight people who eat "too much." Very little is said about the selfishness and self-indulgence involved in a life which makes one's appearance the center of all values, and subordinates all other considerations to it. I do not know how often people are aware of the emotional sacrifice of staying slim. An English writer, Clemence Dane, expressed it succinctly: "Staying slim is like being witty—it is beastly hard work."

Chronic malnutrition based on abnormal preoccupation with weight is common, but not readily recognized as abnormal because it appears under the guise of desirable slimness. These chronic reducers, the "thin fat people," are likely to escape correct diagnosis because our slimness-conscious culture will admire their starved appearance instead of offering them needed help. They come to medical attention only when the weight preoccupation interferes with their living, or when malnutrition gives rise to complaints of fatigue, listlessness, irritability, difficulties in concentration, or chronic depression. It has become customary to prescribe tranquilizers for them; three square meals a day would be a more logical treatment, but one that is equally unacceptable to physicians and patients who share the conviction that being slim is good and healthy in itself.

Frequently these people come to the attention of psychiatrists. Though successful in controlling their weight, they have remained unhappy and dissatisfied, and this theme, with endless variations, runs through their many complaints. Just as food never satisfied them, never gave them what they really wanted, so they are now dissatisfied with their new slim figure and disappointed in what it has achieved for them.

Toby, aged eighteen years, became severely depressed during her senior year in high school. She had always felt that she was destined to lead a lonely life. She was convinced that no man would love her because she was a brilliant student and "too fat." Since the age of fifteen she had been obsessed with dieting. She was tall (5'8") and her weight had never been excessive; 135 pounds had been the highest figure. At times she had forced it down to below 110 pounds. However, this did not relieve her problem; she was acutely unhappy and embarrassed by remarks about her being "too skinny." She also tried to be "like everybody else" by being less conscientious about her school work, but then was distressed when her grades dropped. She tried to participate in social activities and dated a young man who seemed to be in love with her. She had no real feeling for him and became alarmed when she gained some weight during this more relaxed period. Now she missed the remarks about how thin she looked. She became depressed and acutely suicidal, had to interrupt her schooling, and was referred for psychiatric treatment. The obsessive concern with her weight and figure was a camouflage for her deep-seated self-doubt and identity confusion.

Even without such acute disturbance, many are handicapped in their active participation in life. They seem to be successful in controlling their weight but in reality they are crippled in their whole adjustment because they often suffer from nutritional deficiencies and can maintain the low weight only at the sacrifice of mature development.

The case of Beryl is an example that successful reducing in itself does not solve personality problems. She came for psychoanalytic treatment when she was twenty and quite slim, but acutely dissatisfied and depressed. I had first met her when she was sixteen and enormously fat. At that time she had succeeded in getting herself thrown out of a progressive boarding school, having deliberately behaved in a way that even the liberal policies of this school could not tolerate. Her attitude toward her fatness was also defiant. She was quite exhibitionistic and argued that she could be as free with her body and wear the same type of clothes as slim young girls.

Beryl was the youngest daughter of a couple who, after a stormy marriage, had finally separated and gotten a di-

vorce. Her misbehavior at school had been an effort to
force her mother to make a home for the children instead
of sending them to boarding schools. When she came for
treatment when she was twenty years old and in college,
she had lost a considerable amount of weight and now
spoke openly about her former attitude. Weight had been
a problem since she had been about ten, and she had always
been angry about being fat because it had meant "being
inferior. I felt it was like a cross to bear. It is tough to be
born that way. You either practically starve or you gain ten
pounds when you just look at sweet things. It is kind of a
gyp, a lousy break to be born that way."

She was at her fattest when she was sent away from
boarding school. She had never admitted the figure for her
highest weight; it probably was in the neighborhood of 250
pounds. In the intervening years she had traveled a good
deal, and by being careful about what she ate she had
succeeded in holding her weight at about 170 pounds. She
had spent one summer with her father who had formerly
been so cruel about her being fat; she found that they had
many interests in common, and that they were gifted in the
same artistic field. For the first time she felt she was being
valued by her father, and he convinced her that being slimmer would be a great asset for her. She went to a reducing
establishment and forced her weight down to 135 pounds.

Although she now looked beautiful, she was not satisfied: "I want to be underweight so that I can stop worrying
about what I eat. I still cannot eat sweets like ordinary
people. The minute I eat sweets my system craves a lot. I
have to do the one or the other, either diet—or go hog wild
on sweets and all that stuff." She recalled the time she was
at her fattest: "I really did not care about being fat then,
but I did care about people infringing on my rights, on
telling me what to do and what to eat all the time. I know
what to eat and I know what is fattening, but I will not do
it when they keep me on a diet." Her whole concept of
childhood was that it was something that was inflicted on
children. Being fat had been the worst and most painful
experience of this state of helplessness.

Now that she was finally thin and glamorous, she expected that life would compensate her for her past suffering. Most of all she wanted admiration; she did not just want to be liked as an intelligent and pretty young girl, but she wanted special admiration for the fact that she had done it herself, and that she had sacrificed to be beautiful. She also wanted praise, admiration, and spectacular recognition for her intelligence and artistic talents, although she had done nothing to develop them.

At the same time she was disgusted with the overemphasis on looks. "All they care about is looks. I want them to like *me*. I felt lousy the way I looked when I was fat, but then they put *all* the emphasis on looks. Now I have got looks and I know I am right, but I hate people who make comments about it. That shows they don't like *me* for what I am." Yet if a young man did not make a great fuss about her good looks, or did not admire her in an articulate way, she was quite angry.

She developed an exaggerated interest in clothes, showing that she was far from content with her appearance. "I am never satisfied with the way I look. I always keep changing things around me, everything. I change my dress as often as four times a day, and even then I don't like the way I look. I would like to have a different color hair. A girl should not be as tall as I am. I disapprove of everything about myself. Just everything about me is wrong." Or,

When I see a dress in a window, or see another girl has something, I just cannot stand it not to have it. I feel I have to grab it, and I don't care about anything else. I have to buy it. It makes me feel so good, it makes me feel secure, standing there and looking at them—there they are! You can't think about clothes and eating together. If I get clothes, I don't care about eating. They just don't go together. I want my clothes to be special, but I also want to have what other people have. I just want everything. I want the best and the most, and I just love to see a sparkling arrangement of clothes.

One kind of hunger (for clothes and glamour) takes the place of the other hunger (for food). I never understood how women could keep so thin, just having coffee for breakfast.

I always thought they were bitchy women and everybody hated them, but now I want to look glamorous the way they do.

But her desire for food was not gone. She heard about someone who was dying of a chronic disease, and she tried to imagine how she would feel if she had only a short time to live. She had a vision of herself lying in bed and indulging herself. "Then I would do nothing but read and I could eat all the things I am not allowed to eat now—chocolate, cake, and ice cream, and everything as much as I wanted. I just would stay in bed and eat and read. Of course, I would get fat, but I would not mind it. If I was going to die anyhow, at least I could eat, and eat, without worry."

With her craving for attention and admiration her relationships to other people, particularly to young men, were quite unsatisfactory. She always felt that *they* had not lived up to *her* expectations. She was very slow in recognizing how this self-centered need to have *her* wishes fulfilled interfered with all her relationships, even with her long-standing friendships with some girls. This became clear to her when one day she visited her best girl friend who had just gotten a new spring and summer wardrobe. "I envy her because I know that I will never get anywhere near that number. I will get some clothes before I go on vacation, but I'm sure it will never be that number. I am not jealous of Mary in other ways, I wouldn't like to have her parents or even her life particularly, but I want to have her *things.*"

Later at night she could not sleep and she had the impulse to sneak over to her friend's house and steal her clothes, or cut them to pieces so that she would not have them either. She recognized this as vengeful and childish, but also admitted that she was envious of friends who were gifted the way she was gifted. Clarification of the neurotic attitude expressed in this demanding and grasping envy was an important aspect of her treatment, and it was a significant step toward a more mature concept of herself when she began to recognize this.

Quite often continuous preoccupation with weight is recognized only during therapy, without the outer appearance suggesting it. A thirty-five-year-old married woman came for psychoanalytic treatment because she had marital problems and suffered from recurrent depressions and severe anxiety attacks. She was good-looking and well-dressed, and it was obvious that she paid a great deal of attention to her appearance. Her only sister was a well-known dress designer with whom she felt in continuous competition. She had never been fat but was phobic about the possibility of gaining weight. She had a good figure, but when she was depressed she would gain rapidly, as much as ten pounds in a week or two. "During times like that, I eat and eat, though I don't even enjoy it—all kinds of things I don't care for, like bread. Then I feel sick, really nauseated, when I look into the mirror." Since she was young, her concept of beauty was looking like a serpent, long and slim, without any curves; once she had a dress of shimmering silk in which she felt like a serpent. "Sometimes I have the strength to be cautious. Then I can become slim: that shows I am *strong*. I am so pleased then if anyone remarks on how pretty I look. I never know what happens when I suddenly cut loose again: just anything may happen and I have to run into the kitchen and eat."

When she feels fat all over, bursting out of her beautiful clothes, she feels thoroughly ashamed of herself and will decide to diet. The dieting usually starts with a big job of housecleaning. She herself will do the work and feels she does it much better than any cleaning woman would do it; the last thing to be cleaned is the bathroom. Then she takes a bath so that she herself is completely clean and after that the diet begins with three days of complete fasting. After having been so hungry it is easier to stick to a diet; even a plate of salad is enough. She feels much better when dieting; at least in the beginning.

Such episodes are preceded by letting everything get very dirty; only when things are really run down can she do something about it, be it dirt or fat. However thoroughly she cleans, she never has the feeling of being as clean as she should be, nor does she ever feel she is as well-dressed and slim as she would like to appear. When she feels "empty" while fasting, she feels slim even before she has lost weight. She is continuously preoccupied with the impression she makes, but has a compulsion to confess "bad things" about herself. Even as a child, when anybody mentioned something positive about her, she would feel terribly embarrassed. "They say it only to make me feel better." She always felt that she suffered in comparison with other children, and thought she looked "horrible," and "fat" was the word for it. Looking at childhood pictures now, she is amazed how pretty she was, not fat at all. When her breasts developed she felt like the fat lady in the circus, and when she sees pictures of a really fat woman, she has the dreadful feeling, "That's what I look like."

The outstanding emotional tone of her childhood memories is the feeling of envy, that others got more, were loved more, got a better education. As a second daughter she felt at a disadvantage, not getting enough education, not even getting new clothes. Most of all she envied boys because much more was done for them. Being fat reminds her of being feminine; she resents it and becomes depressed and starts an eating binge. She always felt cheated and left out, but most things were outside the reach of her power and she could not alter them but had to suffer in silence. The one great advantage about being fat is that one can do something about it; she can achieve beauty if only she wants to. That's why she gets so exalted if she starves and loses some weight fast; it proves that she has the power to change herself.

Her weight fluctuated between 120 and 130 pounds. When she reached the upper point she would begin her cleaning and fasting rituals. It is possible that without this regimen she might have become quite heavy. Though she had never accumulated the extra weight, she was as preoccupied with her figure and every bite she ate, as if she actually were big and fat.

Not infrequently parents, and also physicians and psychiatrists, reinforce a fat person's unrealistic expectation about what he should weigh. Ingrid, aged twenty years, was referred for consultation by her psychiatrist, who mentioned in the referring letter how "stunning" she had looked when she had brought her weight down to a very low level. She had been successful with reducing while in therapy, but then had suddenly relapsed and was now heavier than at any time before.

Ingrid was the youngest child in a wealthy, achievement- and appearance-conscious family; her mother and older sister were small-boned, slim, and well-dressed. In contrast, Ingrid had been a fat baby and by the time she was a toddler her mother insisted that the pediatrician do something about her weight. He put her on a diet and gave her appetite depressants. Ingrid remained large and heavy as a child, but was continuously pressured to be slimmer; several times she was hospitalized to force her weight down. Like her older siblings she did well in school, but at ten or eleven she had refused to work at all, feeling unable to endure the competition. From then on there were repeated efforts to get her into psychiatric treatment, but she refused to cooperate with any plan.

With adolescence Ingrid became severely preoccupied with her weight. She began to demand that her mother keep no extra food in the house. Gorging herself alternated with bouts of faddish and unrealistic dieting, all to no purpose. She retained good social relations with both boys and girls, but there was no dating. When sixteen or seventeen she became involved with a group of hippies and drug addicts. After a brief period of feeling "accepted" she became frightened about their activities. At this point she asked for psychiatric help. She formed a good relationship with her therapist and quite early in therapy said that she had put herself on a diet, that she had heard people ate as a substitute for love; she felt she was loved and therefore did not need to stuff herself. Whatever the dynamics, at the end of about the first year of treatment she had lost 90 pounds, down from nearly 225 to 135 pounds, and she was beautifully slim. This first weight loss was a relatively slow accomplishment and it was felt at the time to be related to her firm and positive relationship to her therapist. However, in reevaluating this period it appeared that even this first reducing was associated with rather faddish diets and excessive use of amphetamine pills. But Ingrid was still not satisfied at reaching this weight and from then on there were many ups and downs. She would gain as much as thirty or forty pounds in a few weeks but then immediately reduce again. The last impetus for losing was a stay at a famous seaside resort by the whole family. Ingrid wanted to look attractive in a bikini bathing suit and lost about thirty pounds in a very short time, and lost some more while at the resort. When she returned home she was at her lowest weight, nearly 120 pounds. She looked strikingly beautiful and people stared at her on the street. She also received boundless praise from her parents and from her therapist who noted, however, that during this period of forced thinness she was tense and anxious, almost manic. During her hippie period, she had dropped out of school; now she decided to take courses for a high school diploma, and also began ballet dancing and yoga exercises. Suddenly she had many dates, something virtually nonexistent before.

Ingrid maintained her low weight for a few months, but then launched herself upon the most compulsive eating binge of her whole life. Jealousy seemed to be related to the eating problem. Her older sister expected her first child and even before the baby was born Ingrid resented that it might receive more attention than she. She would eat constantly, day and night, and during frequent nocturnal icebox raids would eat absolutely everything edible in the house, so that there was nothing left for anyone else. She would eat to the point of being sick, and when she could no longer eat would throw the remaining food down the incinerator.

Ingrid continued in therapy but now was angry at her therapist for not having cured her. She appeared frightened and severely depressed by the sudden aware- ness that she did not want to be thin, though consciously she insisted that she wanted to lose weight. There was rapid increase in weight and by the time she came for consulta- tion she looked as though she weighed more than 200 pounds; she absolutely refused to go near a scale. However, she did not look as monstrous and grotesque as her par- ents' and therapist's description had suggested. Ingrid was tall and broadly built; she looked massive and too heavy for her frame, but her high weight was not as abnormal as the weight she demanded. She had said that she could not possibly be happy unless she could force her weight down to 115 pounds and keep it at that figure. She reminded me of Binswanger's patient, Ellen West, who complained: "Fate wanted me to be heavy and strong, but I want to be thin and delicate" (2).

In reviewing her life story and her previous treatment experiences, Ingrid felt she had always been under mother's domination, overcontrolled and forced to do things; her only way of asserting herself was saying No. During the consultation she was quite responsive and we focused on the deficits in her concepts of control, psycho- logically and biologically, and on the futility of trying to achieve a better self-concept through the manipulation of her weight. She had proven to herself repeatedly that she could reduce but the effort and tension made it impossible to maintain the weight loss. The same applied to her other efforts to achieve something worthwhile.

Progress in long-standing, fluctuating adolescent obe- sity cannot be measured in terms of weight, but only in terms of overall competence. Better weight regulation becomes possible as a result of better adjustment; it is not a precondition for it. Ingrid absolutely rejected a treatment approach in which weight was not the first consideration. But with such a phobic compulsive preoccupation with weight, the first treatment goal must be correction of the unrealistic expectation. Weight regulation must be seen as a positive achievement after other aspects of coping have been mastered.

To weigh less than is comfortable is an all-American preoccupation. The young, the college crowd, have revived the Roman custom of regurgitation after indulging in large meals. This method has become commonplace. When I first heard about it more than twenty years ago, it was considered unconventional, to say the least. Gloria had been introduced to the method during her second year in college, after she had gained excessively during her first year. To her this seemed the perfect solution to her problem and she brought her weight down from 180 to 115 pounds. When Gloria came for treatment five years after she had begun this routine, her weight was approximately 125 pounds and she was panicky for fear she would grow fat again. Actually she was quite slim, and her preoccupation about fatness was quite unrealistic. She had tried to prove to herself that she had a perfect figure by applying for work as a model; when she was accepted she felt reassured and immediately dropped the plan.

Although Gloria had thus succeeded in creating a perfect figure, her adjustment to life had not only not improved, it had deteriorated to a race between overeating and maintaining the perfect figure. This was the important point: it was proof of her power to defy nature. If she could eat as much as she wanted and still stay thin, then she was doing something nobody else could get away with. She took her weight every morning and when she had gained she would become depressed, unable to do what she had planned for the day, because "her power was slipping." This preoccupation with maintaining the perfect weight was part of her approach to life; she needed to be continuously reassured of "complete perfection in every respect."

Going to college had meant leaving home for the first time. Gloria became preoccupied with the idea of being prominent and popular, and worked hard, "like a politician," during the first month to be well-liked and known by everybody and was chosen president of her dormitory. Once she had accomplished this, her interest in other girls and all activities lagged. She became quite depressed but hid it from everybody in order not to spoil the image of perfection. She overate and gained a considerable amount of weight; from then on fatness became the big obstacle standing in the way of her accomplishing anything. She changed to another college nearer her home; "There too, I majored in being different. If I could not be the best in my work, then I had to be unique in other ways. I just cannot help it, I have this compulsion to be special, and I'll do anything to accomplish it." It was during the second year in college that she was introduced to the "method."

Instead of using it to compensate for an occasional large meal, Gloria made it a routine. She had to eat increasingly larger amounts because it became harder to bring the food up. She gorged herself until her stomach bulged, then she emptied herself and felt relieved. The whole procedure took approximately two hours. She would eat one or more large meals in a restaurant, then have six or eight hamburgers, approximately a quart of ice cream, pounds of chocolate and candy, several quarts of milk, and even then she might find that it was not enough and eat a whole pie or cake in addition. These eating spells took up so much of her time that she could not finish college. She tried several times to work, even for a few hours a day, but was unable to stick to any job.

Nevertheless, she felt a certain triumph in having achieved her goal. She felt reassured about her attractiveness because young men flocked around her, although her need to feel superior and acceptable was not sufficiently appeased by this. She wanted to excel in other respects too; she wanted to do something really big that would make a real impression, something like saving the world and doing good for all oppressed people, or saving and elevating individuals she had met in the course of her many activities. These efforts got her involved in many embarrassing situations. Whenever reassurance about her being superior and perfect was not forthcoming, she would go on an eating spree, as many as three or four on some days. The slightest disregard for her feelings, an unplanned evening, or the fear of not living up to somebody's expectations was enough to provoke this urgent need to eat.

Gloria had recognized the neurotic character of her many activities, and had made several attempts at psychotherapy. Yet each time treatment was terminated for various reasons after four to six months. In the course of her work with me it became apparent that she had used her previous therapists as tools to help her accomplish the godlike perfection which she felt was the true goal of life. Whenever she felt that the therapist was not helping her enough, she would find a plausible reason for breaking off treatment. It was only after this delusional goal had been clarified that a valid treatment relationship could be established.

Even then it took long and painstaking work to help her develop a realistic self-concept. The eating binges gradually diminished in number and lost their specific meaning. Treatment came to an end after she had done well in an interesting job for over a year; she was capable of relationships other than ones that involved her being the goddess adored by slaves. The eating compulsion had diminished considerably, also. Gloria has been married now for over fifteen years to a man who is aware of her old problems and difficulties, and the symptoms have gradually disappeared. She has two children who have not developed any weight or eating problems. She has also been able to put her outgoing interest in others to constructive use in a realistic way.

Though the psychiatric exploration reveals severe underlying psychopathology and an unrealistic approach to life, these women impress the casual observer and their friends and acquaintances as enviably slim, attractive, and interesting. They function in a socially acceptable manner, though under severe tension and strain, and far below the level of their potential abilities. They also differ from those in whom the wish to be thinner and the refusal of food results in anorexia nervosa. The difference is one of degree, insofar as the anorexia nervosa patient continues on the downhill course and aims at a body weight far below normal. There is also a difference in kind: in anorexia nervosa a true misperception of reality takes place; though rational in many respects, the distortions concerning weight and food and the reasons why they must deny themselves are truly delusional. Anorexia nervosa is a rare disease; one may think of it as the end stage of the unrealistic preoccupation with weight and size. Just as only a few of the numerous shy and withdrawn obese adolescents develop into full-blown schizophrenics, so only a few of the countless thin fat people will progress to the malignant state of anorexia nervosa.

It is not always a clear-cut decision whether to assign the diagnosis thin fat or anorexia nervosa to a patient. Pamela, whose mother had developed a severe depression at her birth and had taken no interest in her upbringing, grew up as her older sister's shadow. "I let her speak for me." She measured herself only in terms of her sister's achievements, and the sister had been a brilliant student. When she was fourteen she could no longer keep up the competition. Finally, she refused to go to school. She spent one year moping around the house and had some private instruction. She ate excessively and her weight went up to 165 pounds. When sixteen she was sent to a small boarding school which she hated, "I felt like my inside was torn apart, bit by bit. My eating habit blew up—I was really hooked on stuffing my face and I vomited just by bending over." Pamela finally ran away from this school and did not go back to school at all. In spite of her high intelligence and giftedness in artistic fields, at age twenty-two she had had no vocational training. The idea of competing, of having to face a test, threw her into a panic. Though it is far below her capacities, she supported herself through menial work, choosing nighttime or very early morning hours.

Pamela filled her days with eating binges and throwing up, and by the time I saw her in consultation she had maintained this routine for over six years. Her weight had dropped when she was in boarding school and after she ran away, but not to the level of emaciation observed in anorexia nervosa; she had maintained it at or around 100 pounds. She agreed that this was too thin, but she said she would not want to weigh more because then she would be worried about getting too fat. Pamela also knew that the continuous vomiting played havoc with her electrolytes, that her twitching and muscle cramps were related to this. She willingly took medication to compensate for it. She thus differed from patients with true anorexia nervosa, particularly in not being delusional about her body and its functions, but resembled them insofar as she became increasingly isolated, not participating in any social activities.

The observations reported here run counter to the whole campaign against overweight which, in fact, says exactly the opposite: that reducing is necessary to improve one's physical health, social position, and emotional outlook. These arguments are used daily to convince fat people that they should reduce. It seems to me necessary to point out that a mechanical approach to overweight carries grave mental health hazards. The road of propagating scientific standards of nutrition is littered with landmarks of overly zealous errors and failures. It is my impression that the over-eager propaganda about reducing diets, even though obesity is an abnormal state of nutrition, overlooks a basic human problem, the need for satisfaction of vital needs. "The best women are rich and thin" may be a good slogan for the jet set; it is a potentially dangerous ideal for the ordinary overweight person.

BIBLIOGRAPHY

1. Bellow, S., *Mr. Sammler's Planet*, The Viking Press, New York, 1969.
2. Binswanger, L., Der Fall Ellen West, *Schweiz. Arch. Neurol. Psychiat.*, 54: 69-117, 1944.
3. Heckel, F., *Les grandes et petites obésités*, Mason et Cie, Paris, 1911.

NOTES: WHAT I THINK PUDDING SAYS

by **John Deck**

I have met Felix Prine and I think I shall be able to see the son, Lester, soon!

Yesterday, I went to the farm again and Felix came rolling across the grounds toward me, in his cart, smiling, his jowls shaking, his flesh quivering massively. He wears a straw hat with a very wide brim, curved downward; his pants and shirt are floppy, and the tails of his shirt are loose. His feet and ankles are stuffed into untied high-top tennis shoes.

He is immense and of course thoroughly intimidating. Nonetheless his manner is altogether relaxed. I suppose I had expected the worst and felt safe because there were no dogs, no siren alarms, no caretakers carrying rifles.

"I've seen you around. You aren't from the Farm Labor—"

"No, I'm a student," I said. "I want to do a study on your family."

He smiled. "I don't like students coming around here. But it is a pleasure to see a woman, student or not."

I had not expected his flattery. And I am not sure that flattery was his intention. To be frank, there was something threatening about Mr. Prine. I do not think it was just his size.

He is, though not the tallest, certainly the largest man I have ever seen. I should say *human being* I have ever seen. I had never stood so close to anyone so large.

"I used to be secretary-editor of a newsletter in communications edited by Dr. Malcom." I waited, then continued. "Dr. Malcom passed away about a year ago. He

came out here to Prine Farm and was chased away by dogs
and armed men. He died a day or so later."

"He should have sent you in his place," Mr. Prine said,
struggling to assume an attitude which I suppose was
meant to seem romantic, debonair.

"He did," I said. "I plan to continue his work."

A single narrow wrinkle creased the puffy brow. "I think
I heard about someone. I often miss those chases because
I cannot move as quickly as others. I am ill, of course. We
all are. Some sicker than others. I don't understand why
people from the universities come to make fun of our illness. Are you here to laugh at us too?"

It was so perfect an opening, so complete an advantage.
I almost smiled.

"My dear Mr. Prine," I said, "Is there somewhere that
we can talk? I want to assure you, sir, Dr. Malcom had no
intention of laughing at you. He came, and I am here, to
investigate the so-called Prine Gift."

"So-*called?* Do you know what you're saying? It is a true
thing! My son and daughter both have it."

"I know," I said. "You must excuse me. I've read what
little has been written about your family."

"There's never been a Prine over twelve years old, man
or woman, that weighed less than two hundred pounds."
He sounded almost boastful.

"I'm not interested in what you weigh," I said. "Your
son wrote an essay years ago and it was brought to Dr.
Malcom's attention. It caught his eye, and *ear,* if I may say
so. We study communications—the exchange of information, the way it is transmitted, received, and what is used
as a medium. If you would permit me, Mr. Prine, I think
I could convince you that we do not laugh at unusual characteristics. We will take the Gift as seriously as you do."

He did not believe me. "Attractive women have been
here before. They don't stay."

I was certain that Felix Prine was not flattering me this
time.

"I'll stay, if I am allowed to. I will stay until my work is done," I said.

My name is not well known and in fact I am a novice in the field. Barbara Michaels is listed as secretary-typist, editorial assistant, and copy editor in the last ten issues of the *Quarterly Newsletter of Communications* that Dr. Clyde Malcom so heroically published to an often indifferent community of students and scholars. I am pleased to say that the great man gave me impetus to continue his work. I hope, when I have completed my Master's degree, to begin publishing the *Newsletter* again on a regular basis. I have decided, now that the first foothold on Prine property has been gained, to bring out a special memorial issue at my own expense if the Prine study comes to anything. In it I intend to publish all that is known about the Prines, the Prine Farms, and the "gift" or "curse" of the family.

When I came home this evening I began to make notes on the events of the day. (I will continue to do so.)

Then I went to Dr. Malcom's files. I found Weston's first mention of the Prines in the Spring, 1933, issue of the now defunct *Agronomics of the Southwest*. In an article concerned with crops and water and soil condition, his historic footnote betrays a lapse in discipline of which he must have been ashamed:

"Unfortunately the owners of this excellent acreage have allowed gluttony and a ridiculous story about 'talking food' to addle them. So it was that when I approached them to secure permission to run the regular tests I was driven from the property as a common trespasser."

I calculated swiftly how old Felix Prine was in 1933: a boy still, attending the Teague School in the valley. Perhaps he saw the way in which Weston was dispatched. I imagined torches and guns and the howl of hounds, and recalled how poor Dr. Malcom fared little better, although he came in daylight, thank God.

I have decided that the study, whatever form it takes, will begin with the Weston quote. I will then include the beautiful passage Dr. Malcom left to the world.

"I find in all things inarticulate—all incomprehensible sounds—·if not a voice, at least a challenge to the mind that would offhandedly dismiss them as dumb or meaningless or unimportant. I lift a stone, and in its weight and hardness I feel the aeons of heat and cold, the massive changes the rock has *experienced*. Geologists study the mineral composition of the stone; I listen to it. And I hear in the wind that makes of the earth a throat, a voice box, the infinitesimal whispers of speech so foreign no human mind can penetrate their lexicons for the meaning of a single syllable. Yet it speaks to me.

"Oh, it is a glorious adventure, a constant search for the meaning that comes to us in silence, that is encapsulated and hidden in noise. And when there is intelligence behind the sound, how I rejoice! From every side I encounter pricking mystery. A child's discussion with a pet; the gluttonous farm family's member, incredibly fat, seeming to mumble to its food. Even the inhuman roar of a large cat in a zoo as it attacks its ration of bone and meat. These are not just sounds. I listen and, with luck, learn."

—From *A Listener's Notebook* (unpublished)

Of course, Dr. Malcom never heard a Prine mumble. He permitted himself a liberty there, but I hope to justify him. I hope, in fact, to place the great man in the vanguard of our field with the work I do. I hope to repay him in this way for teaching me to "listen and, with luck, learn."

The third of the key documents for this study, and in many ways the most important, is Lester Prine's schoolboy essay, written when he was twelve and subsequently published in the *Newsletter*. The teacher at the Teague School sent it off to Dr. Malcom as a joke, I'm afraid. But it backfired, as some jokes do. I reprint it here in full, although I am sure it was altered somewhat inasmuch as the original copy came in the mail typed. Grammatically uncertain as the author is, I cannot imagine his mastering the typewriter to the degree indicated.

Lester Prine
9/26/62

A Special Way to Eat

They call me Fatty Prine because I am fat. So is my Dad. Mom isn't because she is nervous. My sister Bonnie also my twin is a lot fatter.

The reason all of us Prine people get so fat is because we grow food right on Prine Farm and it gives the best vegetables in the world. The best pigs and cows and sheep in the world too.

We know special things about growing food. Some of us know special names. Like people think the name of lettus is really lettus but you couldn't write the name of lettus down on this page. If you know the real name, like Bonnie does.

Bonnie eats like anything because she hears special names of food and it is just like music to her. She used to tell me the names but she won't talk much now. I don't hear those names. Dad can't hear them.

We eat a lot because we are food experts. But nobody eats as much as my sister. We are all fat in a special way. Some of us are special people.

I hope to revive Dr. Malcom's spirit, to have him speak through me to the world that so ignored him during his life!

Felix Prine met me at the stone gate to his Prine Farm in a limousine, and I must say he was much, much improved.

He apologized for his behavior on the day previous. He said he was afraid I would not return, and used unpleasantness to shield himself against disappointment. I am impressed by his understanding of psychology and the open and aboveboard manner. As yet I am not too confident of the information I received from him.

We had a brief conversation. For me it was a preliminary investigation. And I have made random notes which will of course need further work. Here then is what I have collected thus far (meanings of a few of the terms are not perfectly clear at this time):

Lester and Bonnie Prine are twins. They are twenty years and two months old. Bonnie was the first to show signs of the Gift. Bonnie toppled five years ago, at about age fifteen. Fifteen is, I think, the normal age for toppling.

Twins are not uncommon in the Prine family, but never has a set of twins been gifted.

Bonnie, from about three or four on, began to show the "classic" development: happy, hungry, never eager to form lasting friendships, never particularly outgoing, spending most of her time in the kitchen with the cook. The young gifted come to the conclusion in early adolescence that there is no place quite so comfortable as the kitchen, no companion so necessary as the cook, no activity so rewarding as eating.

Lester liked people. He was devoted to his parents from the beginning, loved life on the farm and spent hours in the fields and at the pond. He is the first Prine, gifted or not, to show the least interest in athletics. Felix says now that Lester learned to float for all the wrong reasons, but he did learn to float. He was considered normal.

So Lester was sent to school. He went to Teague, a private accredited school in the valley endowed exclusively by his family and attended by his relatives and the children of the farm workers.

It is a first-rate institution which has done much to keep the reputation of Prine Farm high among workers. Not only are the children of stoop labor given an excellent preparatory education but, if their parents have exhibited industry and ambition enough, those children who qualify are sent on to a small private college in the county, also quite dependent on the Prines for a major share of its financial support. (An interesting indication of how the feelings of the workers regarding their employer change can be found in the popularity of a child's song: "Fatty Prine, fat as swine." Heard frequently in grades one to six, it is less common among students after those years, and those who do sing it are likely to be the children of migrant families recently arrived.)

At about fifteen, when Bonnie was toppling, Lester began to spend more and more time in the swimming pool at Teague. Walking into the water, he would roll forward on his face in what is called the dead man's float. Felix was so proud of the accomplishment he didn't question it. Then he discovered that Lester was skipping classes, rising from his seat in the middle of a lecture, rushing off toward the pool.

One day Felix received a call from the headmaster. Lester was in the swimming pool and would not come out, and there was a girl's water-ballet class waiting in the dressing room. Felix left for the school immediately.

"He won't come out, sir. Says he can't stand it."

When Lester saw his father, he stood up, hands over his ears. When he removed one hand to wave, he winced.

"I knew what it was, but I didn't want to believe it," Felix told me, and if the Prine Gift is a blessing, as the Prines themselves insist it is, then I cannot explain the unhappy look on the father's face as he said that.

They were driven to a field of young beans. The windows in the limousine, remote controlled, were closed while they were riding, and Lester was able to take his hands away from his ears. When they stopped, Felix told Lester that he would lower the windows, that he wanted the boy to describe the sound he then heard.

"It's a sweet sound, like a baby laughing. Kind of high. Chee-chee-chee-chee and some other sounds. Pretty."

"It isn't too pretty, is it? You don't want to get too close, do you?"

They were driven to a field of ripe tomatoes. When the car was stopped, the windows lowered, Lester smiled and climbed out of the back seat. He went directly to the nearest vine. He jerked a fruit from the vine, took it to his mouth and, according to his father, did not bite it so much as crush it over his *moving* lips. The juice broke upon his chin and dribbled down over his chest and belly. Talking and eating, the boy stood there and devoured over a half dozen tomatoes.

"I began to cry like a child," Felix said. "You see, I had been wrong. I could do nothing to make him what he was, or what I expected him to be. When a Prine has the Gift he is destined to be the happiest of people. His life is constantly pleasant, perfect. And that is why we are different. We are changed. Fat. Horribly fat! But—"

"You have brown hair and brown eyes for the same reasons you are overweight, Mr. Prine," I said. "You don't curse the color of your eyes and hair because it seems normal to you. But surely obesity is also normal in the family."

He told me I was very kind but that, forgive him, he did not believe I felt that way, not really.

"I am a great big mountain of blubber. All of us are. I admire your courage, Miss Michaels, but I am obnoxious to you."

"No, no," I protested.

He smiled, shook his head. "I don't blame you," he said. "You are confident now. Most people are. But you haven't even met my son. You haven't been near the stone house, seen Bonnie. Others have not been as kindly and pleasant as you. My wife, for example."

I almost gasped. I was appalled by my own thoughtlessness. I suppose I blushed.

"Don't let it bother you," Felix said. "Most of the people who call are astonished I exist. If they get over that, they have trouble believing I could have children. Seldom does anyone ask about the mother of the child—my wife. They are dazzled and confused by what they see."

"What . . . where is your . . . is Mrs. Prine around?" I am trying to re-create my confusion, which was astonishing to me.

"No. I am a widower," he said. "My wife took her own life, at about the time that Bonnie toppled. It is pretty common, really. People from the outside marry Prines because they pity us, or for some reason are attracted to fat people, or because they want control of the farm. Once in a while they love us. But when one of their children actually leaves them to live in the stone house, they usually go away. A few commit suicide."

"But if the children are so happy . . ." I began.

"It is a special kind of happiness," he said. "An awful happiness. You would not find it pleasant."

"I would like to reserve the right to make my own decision about *that*," I said.

"Well, when you feel strong enough," he said, "I will let you see and talk to Lester. You are fortunate that Lester is here and still talking. Because he went to school for several years, he is much more articulate than most of the gifted children. Bonnie quit talking to people when she was ten or eleven."

"I feel strong enough right now to meet your son," I said.

"In time," Felix said. "I will tell you openly, Miss Michaels. I am disappointed by people. They do not understand."

"I shall understand," I said.

"It would be a miracle if you did," he said. He shook his head slowly and a vibration began in the neck and traveled down his chest and arms. As the head swung right and left, these movements started and descended, in the manner ripples start from pebbles dropped in pools. I had never seen anything like it before. The ripples began at the terminus of each swing.

Below are some other remarks he made. I have recalled them while sitting here:

—The Gift is really quite simple. Foodstuffs, all of them, have special names. The gifted say they hear part of the name when hungry. When they eat they say they hear the secret name of the food. It is beautiful. It is like music and something else. If you will pardon me, Miss Michaels, it is something like sexual music. They feel it in the organs.

—It is true that some Prines try to escape the call and most are successful. Cousins have changed their names; an elder brother of mine disappeared under somewhat strange circumstances shortly after the Second War.

—There are Prines in almost all of the professions. Medicine seems the least attractive to us, while teaching and the law are quite to our liking. There are other Prine Farms, in different parts of the country, though they may be operated under different names. We also run cattle and sheep. We are rich and we remain so because we must be rich. We have responsibilities. It is necessary that we be able to protect those who have toppled.

—Lester "hears" food in the fields calling out its name. The closer he comes to the food, the louder it becomes. When he eats the sound is at maximum effectiveness; this does not mean maximum volume. It means that the sound is perfect sensory accompaniment to the food being eaten. You will probably get some of the names from Lester, but I doubt he will be able to explain what they mean to him.

I'm sorry you have to hear this, Miss Michaels. It must be repugnant to you. But to us we are blessed. Gifted. That is our trouble.

Doesn't that offend you, the idea? We think we are important people!

—You, Miss Michaels, are unique. Wives and children, knowing less than you know, have left the farm forever. We are in constant danger of losing our land because we depend on outsiders for our marriages. It seems almost impossible but I, for example, must marry again. Imagine.

(Here, Felix laughed bitterly.)

You have great courage and conviction. I will be sorry when you have finished writing.

(I assured him here that, with his permission, I would like to continue my investigation.)

But you must understand, my dear young woman, that everything I tell you and show you will seem to you a gross distortion, if you will pardon the pun.

(I smiled.)

My wife was strong enough until she saw Bonnie go to the kitchen and spend almost a year there. I tried to convince her that she must face up to the facts. Bonnie's joy is boundless. The gifted Prine is the happiest of creatures. She sat there numb.

Then, foolishly, I took her to the stone house and showed her Uncle Lenox. Actually I only opened the door. After that my wife was never the same.

(I told him I could sympathize with her, though I did not understand what she had seen. Her point of view would of course be far more personal than that of an outsider.)

Do you suppose you would care to visit Bonnie? She's only been in a few years. She's young too, about your age.

(I protested that I was much older than twenty.)

I'm sorry. (He was laughing.) You must understand that I am lonely. I have lost a wife and son recently. I was trying to flatter you, but I'm afraid I do not know how.

(I said I was not unflattered.)

Well, thank you. I want you to see Lester soon, talk to him. I notice that he is less articulate now than he was when he first went to the kitchen. But you will find him informative. Then, if you can, and you mustn't feel you *have* to, I would so much like you to see Bonnie. It would mean something to me, personally. And you would be the first person from off the farm who has seen a toppled Prine.

(The first person, I thought selfishly, I admit. I was filled with eagerness.)

I saw Lester Prine today. In this section I will do my best to repeat what he said. Long ago Dr. Malcom told me that a tape recording is an offense against scholarship because it lulls us into worship for the denotational. I agree, but in talking to Lester Prine I found that I was so terribly aware of my physical surroundings, his presence, and the labored speech and thought of the young man that I could scarcely concentrate on what he said.

Therefore, before I forget it, I mean to strain my mind to get down precisely what he said.

Let me say that we met in a huge kitchen and that he leaned—almost lay—upon a tile-covered table made of brick and that while we talked he was served small individual helpings of food by a cook. He ate and made noises as he ate and said nothing while eating. From small bowls he ate a lettuce salad, Canadian bacon, lima beans, candied yams, and other things.

Here is what he said:

If you aren't a Prine, you can't understand anything and that's all there is to it.

I can give you ideas, but nothing—absolutely nothing—can describe it. It's a miracle! We are miracle people, the miracle family!

Once when we were kids Bonnie and I were playing a game about secrets. And when we played we would whisper to each other. We put our tongues right in each other's ears, and breathed air in, like a big gush of air. That was kind of like how the names of the foods sound. Only the noise is gorgeous.

It wouldn't sound good to you. It's special, still a secret. Ours. It belongs here, to us.

Listen, I liked school. I had fun. The kids called me Fatty, but we've always been called Fatty. Fatty Prine is carved on desks, on trees. But a Fatty Prine bought the desks, planted the trees, and hired the parents of the kids. It didn't bother me.

I studied. I liked animal studies. I heard about evolution just about the time I saw Uncle Lenox and began to understand what it meant that Bonnie had the Gift. I remember that at first I was sort of sick and I didn't want anything to happen to Bonnie and I thought: Maybe we are fish. Maybe that was why I liked to swim. Maybe the Prines were the first humans to keep right on going, see, beyond being like the next guy.

Pardon me. That was a lettuce salad—just lettuce, olive oil and vinegar, with salt and pepper. That seems simple enough, but the real sound of lettuce, the secret name of it, can't be written. If you tried to write it out, you would have to write while you are chewing. There are lots of sounds: the ones your teeth make against the leaves; and each bite has a different sound or name because there is more or less oil, vinegar, salt and pepper, and besides you get a big folded piece of lettuce sometimes and then other times maybe only one small piece or two or three pieces from different leaves. Yes. Each leaf has a different sound.

Of course, the first name is like lettuce, because that is what you see first. When it gets into your mouth, it's a lot of L's, with the L feeling for each leaf, and if the leaf is folded, each fold. Then when you bite, it isn't *let*, it's *leccchhheeeeee-cheeee-cheeee-cheee-chee*. But that isn't right. The sound there goes way up into your ears like a cymbal sound in the Teague marching band. Not too long or loud.

I can't tell you. You get the *cheee-cheee-cheeeyak-cheeyak-cheyak*. Because then your teeth go right through the thickness of the leaves and hit together. First a soft hit, then a harder one, a harder hit.

As the leaves get chewed, the one bite, you swallow, and that is a sound. But maybe before you swallow all the first you start on the second and you swallow little bits of the first.

One high *shosh* for the first bite; then *chosh, chosh, shosh, shoosh, shoosh, shush, shush* as the stuff gets softer. Then *shaagong-guh* for the sound of swallowing lettuce.

I had to say that word, *lettuce*. It's just a word.

Now that is nothing, the sound I just told you, because I left out oil, vinegar, salt and pepper, plus what I know about growing lettuce, the work, the fertilizer, water, sprays, the washing and care (and I know something about oil and vinegar and salt and pepper, too). And there are special feelings from my stomach and intestines when I smell and feel and taste a lettuce salad for the first time.

I suppose I can say anything to you. I suppose I can tell you I feel it right down all the way to my rectum. All the way through. Digestion and everything.

Desserts are not so important to me. Sugar is just sugar, and the way sweets feel, to chew them isn't much fun. I would rather eat a cake that the cook hasn't finished baking, so parts are still wet a little.

Here's something. Meat! Good!

I like the meat when it comes up the best. Pork, I watched pigs grow up. When I could carry things I carried the slops to them. I love their meat the best. I love it best when we have a big piece of their meat and we roast it.

If you bite into the end where it's crispy, the sound is like two sounds: *cheeelll* and *shallah.* You say those two sounds to yourself at the same time and that is the name of the crust. Fat just inside the crust—the crust is *pahl-pahl-pahl-pahl,* but deeper in it is more like *poll-llooll-lloo.* The lean meat is something like *jing* at first, if it is juicy; if it is dry, it is *junnnm.* Of course the name of lean meat changes, and so does the fat's name and the crust's name when you chew it.

You can get crust, fat, juicy lean, and dry lean in one bite, and you can hear all those sounds at once.

But before you hear anything, there would be the sound of a pig's life, too. Some of it is like sniffing when you have a bad cold. Some of it is like clearing your throat.

I can start it for you, give you just the first part, about the dirt: *Ffffferrddrrruukkakakafub, bubba, bulubba, sub-ba, sogglesoggle, keeeble ellebelleel lee blee bleek blek blek.*

That part really is just about mud and soft stuff. It is like when the pig is born from the mother, comes out in the blood and water and things, everything soft and floppy. It doesn't take long to hear it at all. The whole name of the pig, which is a hundred times as long as what I just said, you could hear that starting when you took a piece on your fork and ending when you first heard the sound of the crust or fat or juicy lean.

Pardon me.

At Teague we had a music-appreciation course and we listened to symphonies, each movement, the themes and how they give you different parts added together all over one another.

Eating is like that. The special name for food is just like that. It's like Bonnie's wet tongue when we were playing. But it goes on, it never changes. Oh, it is so sweet.

Every bite I eat is perfect. I used to be hungry when I didn't think I had the Gift. Now it's different. Now I can feel the cook coming over with a new dish. I don't look up. My heart begins to beat fast. I can hardly breathe. But I don't look up. He slides the bowl in front of me and suddenly I see the food. I hear it. I take a bite and say its name! It's mine, *my* food!

Lima beans. The smell, the tougher skin, the mushy center, the butter and pepper, the one that you bite into when the others are chewed, the mixtures of well chewed and partly chewed, the sticky slow way it goes down when you swallow. Everything has a name. And it calls out to you. Beautiful. So beautiful!

And it isn't just lima beans! It's lima beans after another dish. With another dish coming!

The words I have to say to you, the names *you* give foods, they have ugly sounds. They hurt my ears now.

But when I was in school even the true names hurt. I was happy at Teague when I was floating in the pool because then I didn't hear the fruits and vegetables from the fields. The beets ring like bells, and onions have voices like coyotes; onions howl, and beans are like birds.

I didn't think I had the Gift and so I wouldn't listen, and the older I got the more my ears roared and screeched. In the pool I didn't hear anything.

But now I hear from all over the farm.

Bonnie can, and so does Uncle Lenox. Imagine, I felt sorry for Bonnie! I used to go off to school and she would be going from bed to this room. And I would say to myself: She's going to miss a lot. She did, too; she missed everything but the fun. She was having *all* of that.

Oh, I miss Teague, sometimes. I liked Philip Berrigan, the boy that used to help me out of the pool, and Arnold and Armstrong Wylie, the twins. George Halstead, too. He could draw pictures. I miss those guys, but they don't miss me. The best of them thought I was fat and dumb.

I felt bad when I had to quit school, and I felt terrible the day they took Bonnie over to the stone house. But both of them were happy moments, great moments! That was when I was stupid.

Listen, can you understand this? My food sings. Every bite is better than a tongue in the ear.

I'm happy.

It took me all evening to write that. It isn't accurate yet. I have failed.

I am disappointed. Reading it over, you get the impression Lester is only vain. That isn't quite correct.

I mean it seems impossible.

I don't know. Already I've gotten further than Dr. Malcom did. I have new information! I know enough to realize that we are not talking simply about naming food. What Lester did when he ate was hum and make noises chewing. But that is *my* interpretation, and I feel as if I am betraying my opportunities by simplifying. I have a chance now to uncover *startling new things, concepts, experiences,* and I am not sure how to proceed!

I discovered my answer. Felix called and asked me how I was.

"Fine," I said. "Only I'm not sure about how it went with Lester."

"Yes. It's a pity you weren't here earlier, when he was smaller and more sociable. I'm sorry but—"

"I don't suppose I could see him again?" I asked. Felix has his gentlemanly formalities and I get tired of them.

"You could see him anytime when he will allow it. And he'll be tractable for a while longer, I hope. But I thought your time here was limited."

"Well, it is! That's why I'm so anxious," I said, "to get everything right the first time."

"I'm not prying into your personal life, Barbara, but you are always welcome to stay on the farm. Because we automate, we have less help, so there are plenty of empty quarters. And, of course, we can feed you."

I paused to think.

"Of course, you'll want to think it over," he said. "And perhaps you feel you should be less intimate with the sub-ject of your study. I won't press you on it. In fact, I won't mention it again."

"Felix," I said, "your offer is generous." I giggled. "I will tell you if I want to stay."

"Oh, it's nothing," he said. "It's just here. We've got more—well, more than we need."

When he offered room and board I thought he was trying to be kind, perhaps to distract me from my unpleasant interview with his son.

Then I thought: No. It is something else.

I must admit that Lester was fat and that the combination of an extremely fat young man and an ego equally monstrous was beyond my expectations. I had not been prepared, and it took me some time to recover myself. By then Lester had begun to drowse while leaning on the table, and I left.

I will explain just how I feel to Felix tomorrow. Being frank will give him the chance to withdraw his offer. Although it is somewhat expensive to maintain, I think I should have this room to return to after an interview.

Felix is the exact opposite of his son.

Felix called for me today, or had his driver do so. And when I arrived at the farm he joined me in the car and we drove around. He apologized, but not excessively, for needing the entire back seat. The little folding seats are quite comfortable, I find. And it is a pleasure to be able to look at him without seeming to stare. I do not stare. But I sometimes think he thinks I'm staring.

"I thought about offering you a place to live," he said. "But I think it is unfair. My son horrified you yesterday. You probably want to finish this whole business."

I told him frankly that I had not been altogether prepared for Lester.

"But further study will make it worse," he said. "Lester gets—well, bigger and more conceited, all the time. Bigger and happier. He won't leave the kitchen now. The only thing that will force him to leave later is that the cook's presence and the exertion of sitting up distract him from the full enjoyment of the food. That's always the case. Now people talk, pans clang together, and perhaps the odor of several things cooking at once confuses him. He will eventually request to leave."

"And that will be when he topples?"

"Yes," Felix said.

"I suppose the nearer he comes to that, the louder and clearer the names of the foods become," I said.

"Yes," he said.

"I should like to be around when he makes his noises, to see how they change."

"As awful as I look," Felix said, "Lester looks worse. And as disgraceful as he is, he will be horrifying when he has toppled. I don't think you could take it. I don't think anyone who isn't a Prine could stand it."

I said I could stand it.

Felix told his driver to take us by the old stone house.

I had seen it before, from across the pond. It is two stories, large and plain, an L-shaped building. Windows with curtains drawn. It is not sinister in any way. We stopped before it. We sat in the car.

"The underside, the basement," he said, "is filled with a huge kitchen. It connects to all the rooms by dumbwaiters. A chef is at work in the basement at all times, and there are attendants who take dishes from the stoves to the dumbwaiters. Servings arrive at intervals of from ten to twenty minutes depending on the complexity of the dish being prepared."

"How many people live in the house now?" I asked.

"There are, besides Bonnie, five of us in there now. When the four on the top floor quit eating, all the spaces there will be full. Bonnie is the first on the lower floor."

"When they quit eating?"

He looked at me. "We seal the doors," he said.

He shook his head. He gave the driver instructions to return me to my motel. At the door of his house, a modest bungalow directly across the pond from the stone house, he said:

"You are braver by far than most people. But the task you have set for yourself is impossible. Thank you for trying. You have made me feel like a human being these past few days."

He gave me his hand. It was firmer than I expected, and drier. He was sad and lonely and I felt sorry for him.

It is hours later.

I am at the motel now and I have just called Felix. I asked him to send the driver back. I told him I had apostasized myself by not fulfilling my obligations.

"Let me visit Bonnie," I said.

"If you allow yourself to see her," Felix said, "the farm is yours. There will be no secrets."

"I'll do it," I said. "Send the car."

Dr. Malcom, forgive me, but I am frightened. I am trembling.

It is all over and yet it has just started. It is as if my life ended and began in a single moment. I am not the same, but those words above I wrote. These notes are mine. This is my writing.

As you enter, you immediately smell food cooking and hear, faintly, water running.

The stair rises ahead. There are hand-hewn benches and plastered walls without pictures. We turned left.

Bonnie's room was down the hall to the very end. While we walked to it, passing door after door that stood ajar but not opened widely enough to see inside, Felix said:

"We seal them when the dumbwaiters bring back dishes that are not emptied. A great uncle of mine, Elwyn, had his door sealed when I was a boy. My father sealed it. I have done the same a few times. Two cousins and an aunt."

As we approached Bonnie's room, the sound of water flowing grew louder. As we entered I was struck by moist air, warm but not hot, and a louder sound of water, pouring water.

"There is a fountain under here, a perpetual cleansing. I hope such an idea does not offend you. It is necessary."

"Where is she?" I said.

"There," he said. "We are looking at her back. Wait. You'll figure out where you are in just a minute."

There was no recognizable contour, no fold of flesh or structuring that I, with my limited knowledge of anatomy, could recognize. I was about to ask Felix if she were not covered with something when suddenly I heard a mechanical snap and whir. And a huge mass lifted off the top and, while attached, began to weave and circle in the air. At the end of the mass, which again was shapeless, I saw a number of short projections that, to my astonishment, I later realized were fingers. The attached mass was therefore an arm. And it was connected to the body by a shoulder.

"You see?" Felix said. I could recognize the dear man's anxiety. He was terrified that I would turn on him, or run away. Of course I had no intention of doing so.

"The arm moves about after the dumbwaiter goes down; it curves about waiting for the next delivery."

The arm was about as long as a child of, say, two. In some way its bulk suggested a very fat infant trying to dance, though the comparison will serve us no further purpose. It wove about; the fingers fluttered and tremors ran the length of the arm. When it tilted too far to one side or the other, the loose stuff within flowed to the low side, almost as rapidly obedient to the pull of gravity as sand in a bottle.

Now that I saw this substance was an arm, I again looked over the bulk of her and found no anatomical landmark. She gave the impression of something melted. I later discovered that Bonnie lay on her side and that the leg on top had covered the leg beneath. The upper side of the foot had draped fatty tissue over the lower foot. The upper buttock, in this case the right one, had loosened and now it reached the deck beneath her.

By the way, the floor was of tile, sloping gently toward the center, where the flow of water carried off her wastes.

The arm continued to weave until there was another whirring sound, another click. Then, from end to end, the great bulk quivered, and a low, sensuous sound came from the far side. It was a human voice.

"Nahmahnahmahnumanumanumanuma. . . ."

"Something soft. That's the sound she makes for soft," Felix said.

I confess that for a moment there, listening to the diminuendo of her voice, I almost missed what might well prove to be the most important discovery of my life. But my training under Dr. Malcom did not fail me.

"The sound *she* makes. You mean they don't all make the same sound."

"Similar sounds," Felix said. "Lester's soft begins *noomooo* and goes on to *nnnmmmmmmmnnnnmmmmm.*"

Something registered at once. But I confess I was still irrational. Astonished by the huge thing there, I was struggling with a resistant reason that would not accept Bonnie as human.

"I'm sorry," Felix whispered.

And when I could not respond, he said:

"It would be hard for you to do so, but if you could look at her face. It is a face. You can see an eye and a nostril. Then you know."

I nodded. I think I nodded or just walked on. He was ahead of me.

There was a tangle of curly damp hair through which I saw a wild eye and a nostril that seemed unusually big. I thought at first it was the mouth. The whole face reminded me of a photograph I once saw of a whale's head. The head covered the picture from frame to frame, and in the lower right-hand corner was an eye, and only the eye was alive.

This comparison came to me much later, several days later. I am writing this several days later.

Oh, yes, I saw the dumbwaiter, the hand scooping chocolate pudding from the bowl onto the floor just before the heavy cheek. Out from under the cheek came the tongue. It scooped the food in, under the cheek, out of sight.

Her name for pudding continued all around us as she ate.

That's all I have to say right now.

Bonnie's eye did not look at us. Never did she acknowledge our presence if she was aware of it. The water's trickle was slight and clean and remote, and I confess to loving it. I remember how soothing it was, and how enjoyable was the steamy feeling of the air.

When she finished the pudding and replaced the bowl, a jet of water inside the shaft cleansed her fingers. The door snapped shut, an electrical whirring began, and the arm rose, began its trembling dance, the fingers weaving about, and then the eye, staring out of the smooth convexity of the cheek and brow, seemed to roll in its socket with the movement of the arm.

I thought it was time to leave, and we left.

Outside, I felt giddy. I sat first on the bench. But before that I leaned against a wall. Then I sat on the bench.

"You're ill," Felix said. "Stay here and I'll have a car brought around and take you to a doctor."

"I do not need a doctor," I said, still distraught. "I want to sit right here. On this bench. For a minute."

I recall my words clearly and my emphasis.

"You are truly a brave and unusual girl, Barbara," he said.

I did not answer. Something was bothering me.

"You've seen the worst now, you know. Nothing is . . ."

"Please. I'm trying to recall—yes, I know. You said that Lester and Bonnie have different ways of naming, or calling out the name, for something soft like pudding?"

"That's right."

"That's interesting. This is just the kind of discovery I hoped I would make. I find it interesting."

"Good."

"Let's go," I said.

He helped me up. He was stronger than I expected. He did not touch me again, but he opened the door of the stone house for me and then he opened the door of the car.

"If you want to sit in back I can lean against the—"

"No, no, no!" I almost screamed. It was not the first time I had almost screamed since I left the room.

I was glad to be in the car, but when Felix wondered if I wanted to go home, to the motel, I said I didn't think so. In fact, later I asked him to have my things brought to the farm and I stayed here. I have since.

I think I have discovered something very important, but I am not yet sure what it is.

The other night I had some tapioca pudding and I began eating it, and I said *nnnnuuuuunnnggguuunnnnggguuuunnnnggggg* to myself. It seemed to enhance the taste. I'm sure of that. But perhaps I wanted it to, for Felix's sake.

Felix said I can record the sounds Bonnie and Lester make when they are served the same dishes and perhaps I will discover some pattern. If we could formulate the rules that govern the Gift, it would be quite an advance, quite a feather in my cap, professionally speaking. The farm is entirely self-sufficient and has workshops so that such things as plumbing and construction can be done by trusted employees. People are fond of Felix, but I sometimes think they take him for granted. I told him I was going to buy him a handsome big hat some day, a gentleman farmer's hat, to give a little flair to his dress.

Bonnie was, I estimate, four feet across at the top and seven to ten feet at the bottom. Her head was far down from the sort of blunt, rounded-off top of her. You wouldn't say from her shoulders.

Just now I stay away from Bonnie and talk only to Lester. He gets bored and sometimes won't answer, particularly when I ask him to name a dish he isn't eating.

He sometimes cries if the name of it comes to him.

It is incredible. Oh, Dr. Malcom, it is all so incredible!

Felix has also promised to put up the money for a special issue of the *Newsletter*. He has been wonderful in every way. He has shown me the farm, from end to end.

BUSINESS: A SKIRMISH
From THE COMMON HEART

by Paul Horgan

Just before the Harvey House dining-room doors closed for "late," Willa saw the man come in for breakfast, treading heavily on the sunlit floor of the restaurant. He was enormously fat, and walked with his weight poised so that he leaned a little backwards. He was spanked for the morning, with powdery pink jowls, cheeks that dewlapped over one another in tingling splendor. Beautifully groomed, too, a fat man who cherished every inch of his great surface. His eyes were still liquid and blurred from sleep; but so enclosed by the flesh which he put forth that they seemed remote little vials of intelligent blue, lost in that Chinese profusion of curved surface. His movements had something of that spacious and impressive quality to be found in a larger reproduction of something ordinarily familiar on a modest scale. He was captain of an incidental majesty, and moved to his table like the essential half, the completive force, of any whole.

When he sat down, he opened wide his legs, so that his southern hemisphere could depend in space. He set his left hand elegantly tented with spread fingers on his serge thigh, and gazed upon the menu. There was a very special melon announced. He conversed about its promise with Willa and she gave it a fine character. He ordered it.

In the little pause, he looked around, and yearned for newspapers on a near-by table, but let them lie. His neck rolled like a rubber bag full of water over his tight and beautifully pressed collar. His hair was brushed shining flat on his Roman pate.

236

Then Willa started across the room with the melon, and he watched her.

He watched the melon coming toward him, the cool succulent, taste-thrilling sight of it, that pale sparkling heart of fruit, with the chilled lime lying on it to be squeezed. He settled a little nearer the table, and his great pink head moved to follow her as she curved around him to set his fruit down.

And now the morning became spangled and tingling with delight.

He sat so close to the table that he had to look straight down his rolling cheeks to see his plate. This would have buried his little avid eyes in their sacs if he had not raised his eyebrows to stretch his upper lids open so that he had drawn mandarin folds of skin there. His mouth worked slightly open, and appeared to pretaste what he readied.

His whole immense bulking body was intimate and tender with anticipated pleasure. His clean, packed fingers turned the melon and sparkled the lime juice on its every facet, and his lips worked, his cheeks shrunk with tart excitement away from his lips, and his hands were delicate, so fond, in their touch. His tongue was the agent of his hope and want. The taste buds electrified him with the messages he liked best of all in this world to receive. He moved in little pressures against the table, toward his dear melon, that cold and glorious experience at the start of the day.

He had the confidence of the blessed. If after all this it were not a good melon! But he salted it, and the sparkle of the salt and the fragrance it induced from the melon meat could mean only one thing.

He set the plate a trifle away, then, the better to see, and like a pianist serene with arrogant technique let his right paw fall to the silverware where it ever so lightly and surely took up the large spoon.

He moistened his lips.

He opened his mouth, while he spooned out a large and inspiring morsel of the melon, and because his bosom was so vast, his arm had to travel not across it but around it, and the elegance of this arc was like a consummation.

The delicious, dripping moment arrived, and he expressed appreciation in every fine and happy pound of his being.

He took the bite in his mouth, and from his little eyes so genial and so fattened over, there came a tiny stream of appreciation, the fat man's ichor, his thanks for this Thy bounty, and his right thigh trotted ever so slightly on the edge of the chair seat, and the spoon descended for yet another and another scoop of chilled fibrous fruit.

When he had filled his cheeks several times with the luscious grainy meat, so that he was assuaged for a moment, he took a deep breath and turned his attention to Willa, believing that he was doing so without her noticing. He wanted to size her up. Clever thing to do, come here for breakfast first, get 'n impression, make plan, not enough men in bizness took trouble, look ahead, find out class of client got deal with, that was all. He was almost panged by the "pushover" before him. She was little, and gray, and pathetically eager, he felt. A word from whom? from a majestically dissatisfied patron of this dining room, and what? What: out she goes. Power. Big man, Treadwell. Everybody said Treadwell was a shrewd bizness head. Otis L. Treadwell. Name's on m'card, here, in m'inside pocket.—and conversely, a kind word, flattery, and likely the deal was done.

Willa saw him, all right. A salesman type. She knew enough about them. No more morals than an alley cat. *Look out,* she always said, look out for a man who spends so much time on *how he looks,* fat or lean, don't matter, all they want is feed theirself, at somebody else's expense.

She served his breakfast silently and neatly, and when he strode away with the gentle ponderousness of his weight, his arms swinging out from his body because they couldn't hang down, she snipped her nose in the air with her opinion of him, but said again that the public was made up of all kinds, never forget that, she was before the public, and she always felt almost more like an actress than a waitress when she remembered that; a charming dare.

FAT

by **Raymond Carver**

I am sitting over coffee and cigarettes at my friend Rita's and I am telling her about it.

Here is what I tell her:

It's late of a slow Wednesday when Herb seats the fat man in my station.

This fat man is the fattest person I've ever seen, though he is neat appearing and well dressed. Everything about him is big, but it is the fingers I remember best. When I stop at the table near his to see to the old couple, I first notice the fingers. They look three times the size of a normal person's fingers—long, thick, creamy fingers.

I see to my other tables, a party of four businessmen, very demanding, another party of four, three men and a woman, and this old couple. Leander has poured the fat man's water, and I give the fat man plenty of time to make up his mind before going over.

Good evening, I say. May I serve you? Rita, he was big, I mean big.

Good evening, he says. Hello. Yes, he says, I think we're ready to order now.

He has this way of speaking—strange, don't you know. And he makes a little puffing sound every so often.

I think we will begin with a Caesar salad, he says. And then a bowl of soup with some extra bread and butter, if you please. The lamb chops, I believe. And baked potato with sour cream. We'll see about dessert later. Thank you very much, he says, and hands me the menu.

240

God, Rita, but those were fingers.

I hurry away to the kitchen and turn in the order to Rudy, who takes it with a face. You know Rudy. Rudy is that way when he works.

As I come out of the kitchen, Margo, I've told you about Margo? the one who chases Rudy? she says to me, Who's your fat friend? He's really a fatty.

Now that's part of it. I think that's really part of it.

I make the Caesar there at his table, him watching my every move, meanwhile buttering pieces of bread and laying them off to one side, all the time making this puffing noise. Anyway, I'm so keyed up or something I knock over his glass of water.

I'm so sorry, I say. It always happens when you get into a hurry. I'm very sorry. Are you all right? I'll get the boy to clean that up right away, I say.

It's nothing, it's all right, he says, and he puffs. Don't worry about it, we don't mind. He smiles and waves as I go off to get Leander, and when I come back to serve the salad, I see he has eaten all his bread and butter.

A little later when I bring him more bread, he's nearly finished his salad. You know the size of those Caesar salads?

You're very kind, he says. This bread is marvelous.

Thank you, I say.

Well, it's very good, he says, and we mean that. We don't often enjoy bread like this.

Where are you from? I ask him. I don't believe I've seen you before, I say.

He's not the kind of person you'd forget, Rita puts in with a snicker.

Denver, he says.

I don't say anything more on the subject, though I am curious.

Your soup will be along in a few minutes, Sir, I say, and go off to put the finishing touches to my party of businessmen, very demanding.

When I serve his soup, I see the bread has disappeared again. He is just putting the last piece into his mouth.

Believe me, we don't eat like this all the time. He puffs. You'll have to excuse us, he says.

Don't think a thing about it, please. I like to see a man eat and enjoy himself, I say.

I don't know, he says. I guess that's what you'd call it. He puffs. He arranges the napkin. Then he picks up his spoon.

God, he's fat! says Leander.

He can't help it, I say, so shut up.

I put down another basket of bread and more butter. How was the soup? I say.

Thank you. Good. Very good, he says. He wipes his lips and dabs his chin. Do you think it's warm in here, or is it just me? he says.

No, it is warm in here, I say.

Maybe we'll take off our coat, he says.

Go right ahead, I say. A person has to be comfortable.

That's true, he says, that's very, very true.

But I see a little later that he is still wearing his coat.

My large parties are gone now and also the old couple. The place is emptying out. By the time I serve the fat man his chops and baked potato, along with more bread and butter, he is the only one left.

I drop lots of sour cream onto his potato. I sprinkle bacon and chives over his sour cream. I bring him more bread and butter. Is everything all right? I say.

Fine, he says and puffs. Excellent, thank you, he says, and puffs again.

Enjoy your dinner, I say. I raise the lid of his sugar bowl and look in. He nods and keeps looking at me until I move away. I know now I was after something, but I don't know what.

How is old tub-of-guts doing? He's going to run your legs off, says Harriet. You know Harriet.

For dessert, I say to the fat man, there's the Green Lantern Special, which is a chocolate pudding cake with a

special sauce, or cheesecake or vanilla ice cream or pineap-
ple sherbet.

We're not making you late, are we? he says, puffing and
looking concerned.

Not at all, I say. Of course not. Take your time. I'll bring
you more coffee while you make up your mind.

We'll be honest with you, he says, and he moves in the
seat. We would like the special, but we may have a dish of
vanilla ice cream as well. With just a drop of chocolate
sauce if you have any, please. We told you we were hungry,
he says.

I go off to the kitchen to see after his dessert myself, and
Rudy says, Harriet says you got a fat man from the circus
out there. That true? Rudy has his apron and hat off now,
if you see what I mean.

Rudy, he's fat, I say, but that's not the whole story. Rudy
just laughs.

Sounds to me like she's sweet on fat-stuff, he says.

Better watch out, Rudy, says Joanne, who just that minute comes into the kitchen.

I'm getting jealous, Rudy says to her.

I put a big bowl of special in front of the fat man and
the vanilla ice cream with chocolate sauce to the side.

Thank you, he says.

You're very welcome, I say, and a feeling comes over
me.

Believe it or not, he says, we have not always eaten like
this.

Me, I eat and I eat and I can't gain. I'd like to gain, I
say.

No, he says. If we had our choice, no. But there is no
choice. Then he picks up his spoon and eats.

What else? Rita says, lighting one of my cigarettes and
pulling her chair closer to the table. This story's getting
interesting now.

That's it. Nothing else. He eats his desserts, and then
he leaves and then we go home, Rudy and me.

Some fatty, Rudy says, stretching like he does when he's tired. Then he just laughs and goes back to watching the TV.

I put the water on to boil for tea and take a shower. I put my hand on my stomach and wonder what would happen if I had children and one of them turned out to look like that, so fat.

I pour the water in the pot, arrange the cups, the sugar bowl, carton of half and half, and take the tray into Rudy. As if he's been thinking about it, he says, I knew a fat guy once, a couple of fat guys, really fat guys, when I was a kid. They were tubbies, my God. I don't remember their names. Fat, that's the only name this one kid had. We called him Fat, the kid who lived next door to me. He was a neighbor. The other kid came along later. His name was Wobbly. Everybody called him Wobbly except the teachers. Wobbly and Fat. Wish I had their pictures, Rudy says.

I can't think of anything to say, so we drink our tea and pretty soon I get up to go to bed. Rudy gets up too, turns off the TV, locks the front door, and begins unbuttoning his shirt.

I get into bed and move clear over to the edge and lie there on my stomach. But right away as soon as he turns off the light and gets into bed, Rudy begins. I turn on my back and relax some, though it's against my will, but here's the thing, when he gets on me I suddenly feel I'm fat. I feel I am terrifically fat, so fat Rudy is a tiny thing and hardly there at all.

That's a funny story, Rita says, but I can see she doesn't know what to make of it.

I feel depressed, but I won't go into it with her. I've already told her too much.

She sits there waiting, her dainty fingers poking her hair. Waiting for what? I'd like to know.

It is August.

My life is going to change. I feel it.

THE TALE OF SOUPY-KASPAR

by **Dr. Heinrich Hoffmann**
Translated by **Mark Twain**

Young Kaspar he was kernel-sound,
A fleshy cub and barrel-round;
Had cheeks all rosy-red and fresh,
Was fond of soup—it added flesh.
But finally, with scowling brow,
He said he'd strike, and make a row:
"No swill for me; I'm not a cow,
I will not eat it—loathe it now;
I can't! I won't! I shan't, I vow!"

A day rolled slowly o'er his head—
Behold, his flesh began to shed!
Yet still his strike he did maintain,
And screamed as erst with might and main:
"No swill for me; I'm not a cow,
I will not eat it—loathe it now;
I can't! I won't! I shan't, I vow!"

The third day came—lo, once so sleek,
Observe him now, how thin and weak!
Yet still his flag he feebly flew
And hailed that humble dish a-new:
"No swill for me; I'm not a cow,
I will not eat it—loathe it now;
I can't! I won't! I shan't! I vow!"

The fourth day came, and here you see
How doth this little busy bee;
He weighed perhaps a half a pound—
Death came and tucked him in the ground.

DR. NOLEN'S MAGIC BRINGDOWN

by **William A. Nolen, M.D.**

First, the good news: all diets work.

Next, the bad news: none of them work for long.

I have an internist friend who once made a specialty of treating overweight people. He worked hard with and for them—spent endless hours going over their diets in great detail—spent other hours encouraging, cajoling and, when appropriate, even threatening them with the dire consequences he saw in their futures if they failed to lose weight. Over a ten-year period he acquired a huge collection of what he came to call his "fatties."

"It was a lucrative practice," he told me, "but eventually I couldn't stand it. I looked back over ten years of hard work and had to admit it had all been in vain. Ninety percent of the patients I had treated were right back where they started—just as overweight as if they'd never met me. I couldn't get them to leave me so I left them. I moved my practice to another city, and now I limit it to those with heart disease. I still have to keep after my patients about their weight, but at least it isn't the only concern they or I have. I'm a lot happier without all the frustration that comes from treating fat people."

His experience is typical. All the studies which have been done on the long-range effects of dieting show that within a year about ninety percent of those who lose weight on a diet gain it all back.

Why does this happen? Why does Mrs. S——, who worked so hard for six months to bring her dress size down from a 24 to a 14, find herself squeezing back into her old clothes just a year later? Who's to blame?

It isn't the fault of the person who made up the diet. If Mrs. S—— loses thirty pounds in six months by following a magic diet invented by a doctor she'll probably lose thirty more pounds in the next six months if she continues to follow the diet. But of course she won't; why should she? Her goal was to drop from 150 to 120; she's done that and now she's happy. She just wants to stay at 120.

So Mrs. S—— goes off the diet. She isn't going to eat too much, just enough to be comfortable. Enough to hold her weight just where it is. She'll use common sense. She isn't going to have any banana splits, but she is going to allow herself a baked potato or a slice of bread now and then. She's tired of eating two heads of lettuce every day. And as for the three gallons of water she's been imbibing— that is definitely going to cease. She's sick and tired of getting up with a full bladder every three hours all night long. Now, instead of a gallon of water, she'll allow herself one martini—maybe two—in the evening. But no peanuts—definitely!

Mrs. S—— goes back to her idea of eating moderately and, little by little, pound by pound, her weight starts climbing. What she hadn't realized is that when any of us uses good judgment, when we eat enough food to satisfy our appetites and no more, we haven't eaten just enough— we've eaten too much. That little voice that says, "You're full, and it's time now to stop eating," never speaks up until it's too late. Let it be your guide and you'll soon look like a blimp. If you want to stay thin you've got to stay hungry. Six months after Mrs. S—— has quit the doctor's diet she's back at 150. But by now another doctor has published *his* new miracle diet. Mrs. S——, of course, grabs at it, and the cycle repeats itself.

In twelve years of practice I've seen hundreds of patients—and friends—bounce up and down, weightwise, as the new diets come and go. We've lived through the Quick Weight Loss Diet, the Calories Don't Count Diet, the Drinking Man's Diet, the Dozen Eggs A Day Diet, the Lettuce Lover's Diet, the Five Gallons of Water A Day Diet, and we're currently living through—or, hopefully, will live through—Dr. Atkins and his Diet Revolution. At least once every year a new fad diet sweeps the country, with the usual short-term results. I've become very cynical. When a patient says, "Can you recommend a diet for me? I'm determined to lose twenty pounds," I cooperate. I tell her all I know about dieting and send her off with one of those little booklets that tells you how many calories there are in a stalk of asparagus. I give her an appointment to check back with me in a month. If she has lost weight, she'll keep the appointment; if she hasn't, she'll cancel. If she keeps losing weight I'll see her every month for six months. After that, as I've already mentioned, she won't be back. She'll be off her diet, her weight will be on its way back up, and she'll be too embarrassed to come in. That's the way, almost without exception, it always goes.

Now, if you'll bear with me for a few minutes, I'd like to review some of the fundamental facts of dieting. Because there are so many people desperate to lose weight I could probably put these fundamentals into a book, call it *Dr. Nolen's Magic Formula for Shedding Fat,* and make a million dollars. But I haven't the heart—no one is going to derive any long-range benefit from this guide. The doctor who sells "miracle" diets is as unscrupulous as one who sells cancer cures.

The first of these fundamentals is one you've heard denied hundreds of times. Nevertheless it remains true and is the cornerstone on which all successful diets are constructed. Stated simply: calories *do* count. In fact, calories are about all that count. If you take in more calories in twenty-four hours than you burn up in twenty-four hours, you'll gain weight. If you take in fewer calories than you burn up, you'll lose weight. There is no way to get around this sad fact: it is a fundamental law of nutrition.

Calories come from food and food, like Gaul, is divided into three parts: fat, protein, carbohydrates. Lean meat, for example, is mostly protein; sugar is pure carbohydrate;

fat—well, you know what fat is, the white greasy stuff on the outside of the steak. When "burned" in the body, one gram of fat yields 9.3 calories, a gram of protein produces 4.5 calories, and there are 4.5 calories in a gram of carbohydrate. A gram—if you're interested—is .002 pounds.

Each of us uses up a certain number of calories every day. How many calories we burn depends chiefly but not entirely on how we spend our time. The man who works eight hours a day as a lumberjack may burn up 5000 calories in twenty-four hours. The man who rides to work in a car and spends all day at his desk may burn only 2000 calories. But you probably know all this.

What you may not know, but probably suspect, is that two men (or women) who do about the same amount of work each day may burn up different quantities of calories. This is because there are individual variations in metabolism (metabolism being the term we use to denote the building up and tearing down of our body tissues, both of which processes go on continually). We all know people who never seem to gain any weight, no matter how much they eat. One of my partners, for example, wanders into my office almost every day munching on gooey pastry— cream-filled chocolate doughnuts are his favorite—two hours after he has had bacon, eggs, toast and coffee for breakfast. He eats all day and he never gains an ounce. If I ate what he eats I'd weigh three hundred pounds in a month. But he's just one of those lucky people whose bodies, for some still obscure reason, burn up an enormous number of calories.

On the other hand I'd like to have a dime for every person who has told me, "Everything I eat turns to fat. I swear I'm practically starving myself, and still I gain weight." Most of the time these people are lying—to themselves and to me; they're forgetting the martinis or milk shakes they drink. But some of them are being honest; they just don't burn up as many calories as I'd expect them to burn, which is most unfortunate for them.

I'd better make it clear here that these differences in individual metabolism are not due, as far as anyone can tell, to glandular disease. Patients always wonder whether their weight gain can be explained on the basis of a "low thyroid." They'd love to find that they can trim down simply by taking one or two thyroid pills a day. Sadly, this is almost never the case. Malfunctioning glands are very, very rarely the cause of weight problems.

Now back to "Dr. Nolen's Magic Formula." Once you assume that calories do count, the answer to your weight problem becomes apparent. Every day you have to eat and drink food that contains fewer calories than you burn in that twenty-four-hour period. If, for example, you take in 2000 calories and burn up 3000 calories, then the extra 1000 calories you burn will come from other tissues in your body—and as long as you have supplies of fat stored away, that's where the extra calories will come from. Every day that you run a 1000-calorie deficit, you'll lose 1000 calories worth of tissue and your weight will go down.

How, with the individual variations we admit exist, can you tell how many calories you can afford to take in each day? The easiest system is just to go on a 1000- or 1500-calorie diet—even the most sedentary person will usually burn up 1800 calories in a day. But there's another system I recommend which, for the short time a patient uses it, seems to work reasonably well.

When I first see a patient I tell him to eat for the next three days just as he has been eating and to write down everything—and I mean *everything*—that he takes in. Count the drinks, the peanuts, the hors d'oeuvres. Then get out the calorie book and see what the average daily calorie intake is. Whatever it comes to, whether it's 1500 or 5000, it is obviously too much, since on that diet he's either gaining weight or staying at a level he doesn't like. I then tell him to devise, using his calorie guidebook, a menu that will reduce his calorie intake by fifty percent or, if he's in a big hurry, by two thirds. If he follows this procedure, he can't miss.

There are a couple of other points I make, since I don't want anyone suing me because they've followed my instructions and acquired a flagrant case of scurvy or beriberi. I tell my patients to be sure to take in at least 100 grams of carbohydrate, 100 grams of fat and 50 grams of protein every day. The body seems to need these to function properly. If they just keep a reasonable balance in their diet they won't have any problems with malnutrition or avitaminosis, but if they want to play it safe they can take one—I said ONE—vitamin tablet a day. An excessive intake of vitamins can—not often, but occasionally—cause medical problems.

I also tell my patients that if they're hungry while they're on their diet, and the chances are they will be, there are lots of bulky foods—lettuce and celery being two well-known examples—which contain practically no calories and will serve to keep their stomachs full. After a while some people will get used to smaller meals and not feel hungry, but, unfortunately, most never get used to the reduced food intake. To get and stay thin, they're going to have to get used to feeling hungry for the rest of their lives.

One question I frequently hear—as you might suspect—is, "Can you give me a pill to help me get started? Once I'm on the diet I'm sure I can get along, but I'd really like some help to get going."

I avoid drugs, such as thyroid, designed to speed up metabolism. I prescribe amphetamines only rarely, and only to those patients who are of unquestionable emotional stability. In fact, I prefer not to prescribe any pills at all. But, if I think the whole venture is hopeless without it, I will occasionally prescribe Tenuate (diethylpropion hydrochloride), a drug which effectively diminishes appetite. As with any drug there are certain precautions that should be observed—Tenuate, for example, should be used with great caution, if at all, by patients who have severe high blood pressure. Generally speaking, however, it's a safe, reasonably effective medication, and not likely to kill anyone or turn him into an addict. Even so I stipulate at the time I write the prescription that I'll only prescribe a ten-day supply and that there will be no refills. After ten days willpower has to take over.

Now, finally, a few words about "fad" diets.

When I started this article I planned to discuss all the fad diets of the last ten years, compare them, and make whatever recommendations or denunciations I thought appropriate. This turned out to be an impractical, impossible idea. There have been too many such diets; more than thirty diet articles get into the general-circulation magazines every year. Recent gems include the Nine Day Wonder Diet, *Vogue's* Super Diet, the Ice Cream Diet, the Eggnog Diet, the Nibbler's Diet, the Sweet Tooth Diet, the Secret Summer Diet, the Yardstick Diet, the Expense Account Diet, the Lollipop Diet, the On and Off Diet, the Keep Your Husband Diet, and the Perfect Diet. I couldn't possibly write a detailed commentary and evaluation of each. But I can give you an overview, which is simply this:

All reducing diets, fad or scientific, have the same ultimate goal: a reduction in caloric intake. Few of the fad diets come right out and say this, of course—most dieters would realize immediately that the diet was going to require willpower, dedication and, most painful of all, some hunger. Fat people want to lose weight, but they don't want to suffer.

So instead, the fad diets accentuate the positive: the food they allow, like steak three times a day or all the cottage cheese you can eat. They do this so that the dieter won't realize that he's actually being asked to cut down on calories. It won't be until the third or fourth day of his diet, when he suddenly realizes he doesn't want another steak or bowl of cottage cheese, that the dieter will realize the regimen isn't going to be any easier than previous ones he's tried. Fad diets work because too much of any one food reduces the appetite. Most fad diets depend on this for their success.

Are fad diets harmful? Usually not—though there are obvious exceptions. For example, the Drinking Man's Diet, which allows you as much booze as you wish but little food—an unofficial but very popular diet, I might add—would not be the optimum diet for a reformed alcoholic. And the A.M.A. seems to have some serious reservations about Dr. Atkins' diet.

Perhaps, since Dr. Atkins' book and, presumably, his diet have achieved such extensive popularity, we ought to consider their defects in more detail. With the A.M.A. and a number of disgruntled patients breathing down his neck Atkins hardly needs anyone else sniping at him; but perhaps he won't think me too unkind if I simply mention a couple of the arguments others have used to attack his diet.

First, it's basically a high-cholesterol diet. Dr. Atkins says that as long as you take in few or no carbohydrates, you can eat virtually anything else you want including large quantities of fat. Fats are rich in cholesterol and many nutritionists feel that high-cholesterol diets are potentially very dangerous. For example, statistics show that individuals who have a blood-cholesterol level above 250 mgms. per 100 cubic centimeters have three times as great a chance of dying of a heart attack as those with a blood-cholesterol below 150. Certainly if you're susceptible to coronary artery disease—and who isn't?—it would seem best to adopt Dr. Atkins' diet very cautiously.

A second hazard associated with Dr. Atkins' diet is the possibility of getting into trouble with gout or kidney disease. When our bodies burn large quantities of fat we get into a state called "ketosis," ketones being end products of fat metabolism. Ketosis leads to excessive retention of uric acid, and uric acid can produce gout and/or kidney trouble. A few days of mild ketosis won't hurt, but a long run of ketosis—and the goal of Dr. Atkins' diet is supposedly "staying thin forever"—could be dangerous.

Diabetics on insulin will have to be very careful with Doctor Atkins' diet. A drastic reduction in carbohydrate intake requires a revision of insulin dosage and, as any diabetic knows, adjusting insulin dosage is a risky business. And since insulin-dependent diabetics are normally susceptible to ketosis anyway, Dr. Atkins' ketogenic diet may aggravate that predisposition.

Finally, Dr. Atkins doesn't have studies to prove his diet works. His "evidence" takes the form of "testimonials" from grateful patients. That sort of "evidence" is no evidence at all; testimonials are easy to come by and are of no scientific value. For all anyone can tell there may be ten fat, Atkins-treated patients for every thin one. All things considered, Dr. Atkins' diet seems a very good one to avoid.

Generally speaking, most doctors don't care what diet the patient follows as long as he follows one of them. The primary goal is to lose excess poundage; how that's accomplished is of minor, secondary interest.

Here is a quote from an article on obesity by George Mann (Sc.D. M.D., Associate Professor of Biochemistry and Medicine, Vanderbilt University School of Medicine) which rather neatly sums up medical opinion on fad diets. The article is in the 1972 *Current Therapy:*

"There is no particular dietary mixture that either makes a man lose weight or is more comfortable for him while he loses. Nevertheless, an endless array of 'reducing' diets intrigues the clubs and hair-dryer lines—and enriches the publishers. These 'reducing diets' have become a large industry . . . serving writers and publishers who prey on the gullible and too often using the approval of unwitting physicians."

The only word with which I disagree is "unwitting."

Do you find this article depressing? I do (and that's bad—maybe you shouldn't be reading it because depressed people often tend to overeat and get fat). But if you're not yet in tears let me now administer the coup de grace.

There is some new scientific evidence which seems to suggest that when you're fat you're fat, even when you're skinny. Medical studies have shown that people who are fat are that way because of the number of cells which develop during childhood. They have more and larger fat cells than thin people. Even if these fat people work very hard and trim down they will not become thin people but thin fat people. Their fat cells may be down but they're not out, and they lie in wait ready to pounce on the first pat of butter that comes their way. Neither Dr. Stillman, Dr. Atkins, nor anyone else can transform a naturally fat person into a thin one.

One final note designed to keep all us fatties from committing hara-kiri. The last line in Dr. Mann's article on obesity reads: "Hippocrates Aphorism no. 35: 'Those do best who are a little fat about the belly. It is bad to be thin and wasted there.'"

Hippocrates, we thank you.

REELY FAT

by *Jeanine Basinger*

Whenever true film fans get together, there is always that special time reserved for eating too much buttered popcorn and remembering favorite fat people on film. It seems that all the movie-going world loves a fat fellow, although favorites naturally vary. From Charles Laughton to Sydney Greenstreet to Laird Cregar to Victor Buono and onward—everyone has his own particular pet and no actor is too obscure to be remembered. (I once listened to a heated argument over whether Harry Holman would have been a better fat Santa Claus in *Babes In Toyland* than Ferdinand Munier. And if you know who either Holman or Munier are, you can cash in your chips right here.)

Fat movie-people lovers usually are divided into two simple categories: those who love fat villains and those who love fat comics. For it does seem that the fat man on screen is mostly one or the other. He is never just an average normal overweight overeater like you and me. He is either a subject of fleshly terror or the victim of a banana peel (two banana peels?).

I personally am partial to fat villains. Maybe it's because I myself like to eat, and I therefore secretly love to see fat people get punished (as all villains do) for having had all that fun gorging themselves on exotic fare. Or maybe it's because I am so terrified of getting magnificently overweight that just the sight of a fat man scares me. Or maybe my mother was frightened by an old Vernon Dent movie. At any rate, I take fat villains very seriously. I have just always assumed that anyone who would get that gross is capable of almost anything awful.

As a little girl, I became aware that fat villains were associated with sexual revulsion. Technicolor princesses were always being warned that, as a fate worse than death, they must marry fat caliphs. Unless, of course, the skinny prince-in-disguise could jump out of that oil cask in the nick of time. Since the prince *was* so skinny (they were all 4-F in those days), he naturally had no trouble getting in that cask in the first place, much less getting out of it. (I always considered this information of great value: if you needed to hide in an oil cask, you had to be able to get in and out of the damn thing. This knowledge cut down my childhood jujube consumption considerably.) There was also the hint of perversion under the surface of the fat man's bland exterior—the assumption being that since his gullet wasn't satisfied with one simple peach, his libido wouldn't be either.

Consider the roster of famous screen villains of ample proportions. Number one ton for most people is the "fat man" himself, Sydney Greenstreet. Greenstreet, a Shakespearean actor who didn't make his first film until he was 61 years old, became the yardstick (the bushel and a peck?) by which other fat villains were measured. The definitive Greenstreet performance, which was, in fact, his first on film, was as the mockingly menacing Gutman in Huston's *Maltese Falcon*. Despite the fact that Greenstreet played in twenty-four movies, out of which only eleven of his roles could be actually considered villainous, he remains forever associated in people's minds with a Gutman-like character.

The Greenstreet villain was a man who seldom did his own dirty work. He had a selection of thinner meanies who did that for him. He did, of course, swat his own flies . . . and he was once seen to deliver vicious blows with his cane to the prostrate body of Humphrey Bogart . . . but only after a henchman had already knocked Bogart out cold.

Film historian William K. Everson delights in the pleasures of watching the inspired pairing-in-villainy of Greenstreet and Peter Lorre. (Everson describes them as an "unholy Laurel and Hardy.") The two together *are* wonderful, but I think I prefer my Greenstreet straight: blank of expression, urbane in manner, calm in danger, bursting out with an insane and unexpected gargle of a laugh . . . or, best of all, snarling at Joan Crawford just before she shoots him, "I should have spit you out the first time you got between my teeth." Obviously, the perfect gourmet metaphor for a fat villain.

A sort of poor man's Sydney Greenstreet, Dan Seymour was evidently promoted from his job as doorman at Rick's in Casablanca just in time to play the police captain in *To Have And Have Not*. Although Seymour resembled Greenstreet physically, he had no real villainous style of his own and inevitably ended up at the bottom of the heap. Instead of imitating Greenstreet on his own level, Seymour found himself satirizing all fat villains in the Marx Brothers film, *A Night in Casablanca*.

A British fore-runner to Greenstreet is the marvelous Francis L. Sullivan. He was at his unctuous best as Pothinus in Pascal's lavish production of Shaw's *Caesar And Cleopatra*. His work in that film inspired me to write my sixth grade "project report" on ancient Egypt. (That may seem odd to some people, but I also was inspired to study astronomy by a Wonder Woman comic book. And my total knowledge of the crusades stems from the passion for research on the subject generated by Henry Wilcoxon's kissing Loretta Young in the reissue of that epic.)

I liked Laird Cregar, too, at least what I saw of him. I had to appreciate him mostly from the lobby cards as my mother wouldn't let me see him as Jack the Ripper. But I loved his suave, elegantly dressed devil in *Heaven Can Wait*, and I caught him on the late show, madly composing a concerto while the house on Hangover Square burned down around his ears. (Cregar died just after completing that role, at age twenty-eight. His death was a great loss to all appreciators of fat actors everywhere.)

Today's most suitable successor to Greenstreet is probably Victor Buono, who, before playing a grim strangler, had to first pay his dues by being himself menaced by Bette Davis in *Whatever Happened To Baby Jane?* The assumption there, no doubt, was that any actor facing up to Davis in that make-up could go on to a superb career in scaring people.

And there are plenty of other fat villains to remember. There's Peter Ustinov as Nero, weeping into his lachrymatory from the Metro prop department . . . and Rod Steiger strangling all the women he can get his hands on . . . and Thomas Gomez and Kewpie Morgan and Raymond Burr and Sebastian Cabot and Oscar Homolka and Peter Bull and Zero Mostel. And, as a fat villain set to music, Walter Slezak as "black Mack . . . of the Caribbean . . . or Car-rib-eeeeeee-an Sea." Mack the Black Moccoco, from *The Pirate.*

And what about Orson Welles, who is positively disgusting in *Touch of Evil?* Surely that scene when a black-wigged Marlene Dietrich looks him over and says, "you're a mess, honey" must stand as one of the screen's really great "fat moments." (Speaking of fat moments, where does Alfred Hitchcock fit into all of this, by the way?)

There is always a group of character actors that some fans say are legitimate fats and others say simply don't have the girth to qualify. These include Wallace and Noah Beery, Erich von Stroheim, Telly Savalas, Akim Tamiroff, Gert Frobe, Leo McKern, and Ernest Borgnine (that big rat . . . picking on a little guy like Frank Sinatra).

On the other side of the scale to all this are the fat comics. Most people immediately think of Oliver Hardy or lesser lights such as Fatty Arbuckle and John Bunny. There's also Andy Devine, of the lovable sidekick school, not to mention Billy Gilbert, Lennox Paul, Billy House, Grady Sutton, and Curly of *The Three Stooges.* Lou Costello was the most popular fat comic of my own youth. Although he was not one of my childhood favorites, I, youthful critic that I was, did point out to my peers that Costello's art was far superior to that of the aforementioned Curly. Walter Slezak and Zero Mostel are known to some film-goers mainly as comics, not villains, and can be counted fairly in both camps. Hugh Griffith had a great role roistering fatly on top of various females in *Tom Jones*, and gravelly voiced Eugene Pallette provided many wonderful moments in scores of good thirties comedies. One of my personal favorites is the unforgettable Robert Morley, destroying a certain kind of pompous intellectual theater forever with his reading of "follow the turtle to my father's tomb" in a seldom-seen British comedy, *The Final Test.*

Some heavy-set actors can't be easily categorized as specifically villainous or specifically comic. Edward Arnold, for instance, made a career out of playing corrupt American businessmen (or politicians). But Arnold also played sympathetic roles, even romantic heroes, a feat attributed by most fans to his genuinely soothing, rich voice, which could be used as an instrument of threat or love equally well. Arnold had the further distinction of playing the screen's first Nero Wolfe. The role was also played by Walter Connolly, another sometimes-good, sometimes-bad fat man of the screen. (Whether Connolly was bad or good, he was always crabby, however.)

Charles Laughton was one of the best and most versatile fat actors in terms of switching from bad man to good man and back. My favorite Laughton bad-man role is when he threatens the outrageous Tallulah Bankhead with this sadistic warning: "I'm going to kill you . . . but I can wait." (I, on the other hand, could hardly wait at all.) As to my favorite Laughton good-guy moment (and, incidentally, one of my all-time favorite film moments in general)—what else but the delicious scene in which he takes a long walk to deliver a very elegant raspberry to his boss—the only "dialogue" in the entire Laughton segment of *If I Had A Million.*

Perhaps the height (or depth) of fat comics on screen took place early on in film history, with the silent comedy series known as *Ton of Fun,* starring The Three Fatties in nothing but a series of comic pratfalls. I am mercifully grateful that I was not around to see these obese beauties doing their stuff.

So far, not much has been said about fat women on screen, and for very good reason. There just aren't too many of them. Fat women are usually on screen just for a sight gag, and are often nameless minor characters good for a joke and not much else. Queen of the fat ladies of film, however, if there is one, might be Marie Dressler, who even had the distinction of appearing in a film called *Reducing.* Or perhaps it might be the indestructible Hope Emerson, whose great film moment comes when she confidently lifts Spencer Tracy over her head with one arm in *Adam's Rib.*

As to other fat women? Well, some people count Kate Smith, but she was never really a movie personage. There were always those heavy-set black maids: Hattie McDaniel, Louise Beavers, and Aunt Jemima. And a whole list of wonderful plump matronly types: Florence Bates, Madge Blake, Marjorie Bennett, and a heavy old ladies list which includes Jessie Ralph, May Robson, Laura Hope Crews, etc.

Two standouts for female comedy figures are the fabulous Babe London, who plays Oliver Hardy's fiancée, and good old Jody Gilbert, that marvelous mountain of flesh to whom W. C. Fields whines in *Never Give A Sucker An Even Break* . . . "I didn't make disparaging remarks about your steak. I merely said I hadn't seen that old horse you used to keep outside around here lately."

And, I suppose, just to be thorough, one ought to at least mention Spanky McFarland, as the official representative of the overweight underage set.

No evening of popcorn and fat talk ever ends without people turning to the subject of which movies are fat. Some movies, you know, really are themselves fat. For instance, *Land Of The Pharaohs* is a lean epic, but *The Egyptian* is fat. *Bringing Up Baby* is a downright svelte comedy, but *Will Success Spoil Rock Hunter?* is, while not really fat, at least a trifle plump. *Scaramouche* (the fifties version) is a greyhound of a costume drama, but *Beau Brummel* (from the same period) is overweight. And so it goes.

I like to have the last word on these evenings of fat talk, with my own particular contribution. My years of working in a movie theater taught me something about the audience's feelings about eating and viewing films. Not only how much would be bought and eaten, but what type of food, depended on what was showing. A love story always increased the sale of chocolate bars. *Love Is A Many Splendored Thing* must have sent Hershey stock soaring. There's something about all that goo on the screen that inspires a desperate urge in the audience for a similar kind of goo on their faces (not to mention the seats). Deep, lasting love and romance kicked off a human need that kept the candy sellers hopping.

Horror films, on the other hand, sent food sales plunging to near zero. How could anyone who was going in to watch a vampire movie be sinking their teeth into something soft while up there on the big screen the scaries were sinking their teeth into something equally soft? (There were, however, always a few strange people who showed up only for horror films. THEY always bought that string licorice and tore at it savagely while the things from another world menaced the rest of us.)

In comedies, people ate lots of popcorn. In adventure films, especially desert epics, they drank lots of Cokes. If the hero or leading lady died at the end of the picture, scads of half-eaten, abandoned goodies would be left in the theater. And, finally, just let a fat woman appear anywhere anytime on the screen, and everyone automatically stopped eating.

But whether you were eating while watching them on-screen or they were eating offscreen to be fat enough for you onscreen, the reely fat people were a joy to behold. Here's to them forever! And pass the buttered popcorn.

I DREAMED I WAS JUNG LAST NIGHT . . .

by *Brian W. Aldiss*

"**I** dreamed I was Jung last night," said Saul Betatrom heavily over breakfast, showing his long eyelashes to his current mistress as he poured cream over his jam puff.

"My, what fun!" Paidie exclaimed boredly. She was tired of his eyelashes. She wanted to go shopping in the bazaar, not sit or lie with Saul all the time; this Indian holiday was getting to be a real freak-out.

"Yeah, I was old Carl Jung, beard and all," said Saul, whipping up the mixture on his plate and spooning it towards his ample lips. "Boy, there I was in some damned church or something in Switzerland, and this trapdoor opened at my feet—"

"Was I there, Sauly?"

"No, you weren't there. I was alone, all by myself, wearing this black robe, see, and I'd just formulated the concepts of psycho-analytic theory, and then this hole opened right up at my feet . . ."

Her interest ceased when she learned that she was excluded from the dream. Hazy memories of other lovers and sexual gymnasts floated into her mind; she couldn't recall a one of them that had ever dreamed of her. She looked over the balcony at the bone-white beach, the line of canted palms, and the ocean. Paidie told herself how much this was all costing Saul, and tried to feel enjoyment.

". . . And there at the bottom of the lowest cellar was a couple of skulls, sort of mouldering and indistinct . . ." Saul was saying. He was head of the New York branch of Zadar Smith World; suddenly recollecting the fact, he piled on more cream and added sugar to the puff. The turbaned waiter appeared, silent at his elbow, and refilled his cup from a silver coffee pot.

". . . Although I'd climbed down so far, somehow I couldn't bend down to reach those skulls. Now wasn't that a funny thing?" He stopped munching for a moment in order to recollect its funniness in tranquillity.

"Yeah, crazy, say, are we going down the bazaar today, Sauly?"

Licking his spoon, he gave Paidie a heavy stare. "They got riots in Kerala, one mile down the road, you know that? The manager says it ain't safe outside the holiday strip. You saw the newscast same as I did, Paidie."

"Oh, Saul, let's go see the bazaar! I want to get outside the strip today. We can take a cab, can't we?"

"We'll see." Women never listened to you, he thought. They were okay but they didn't listen. You could pay men to listen to you, but you couldn't pay women to listen to you. Might be an idea worth developing there . . . He switched on one of the rings on his finger and said into it, "You can pay men to listen to what you say but you can't pay women to listen to what you say." Must be a way of cashing in on a thought like that.

"I listen to what you say, Sauly," Paidie said. "I just want to go to the bazaar. We can't sit here *eating* all day, can we?"

They collected their gear, put on dark glasses and refrigerator hats and drifted through the foyer of the hotel. On the way, Saul tossed down a few dollars (the Luxor Hotel had no nonsense with rupees) and picked up a leg of chicken from a spit to chew.

He was lean, with a flat stomach—fine hunk of masculine body, she had to admit. "I don't know how you keep your figure, Saul. Why you eat just about all the time and you hardly have no tummy at all to speak of. Me, I just diet and diet, yet look at the size of my thighs!" She knew they were worth looking at.

Chewing, he slouched out into the sun, stood gazing across the immense spread of the Arabian Ocean. He meditated on whether to bother answering her, slewing his eyes round as he did so, taking in the scene.

The great hotel sprang up out of the sand like a fortress, its array of bulging balconies like gun-turrets that ceaselessly watched the sea. Coloured umbrellas on the balconies, gay as death, waited to gun down the setting sun.

The Luxor was inviolate, an implacable holiday-annihilator. Round it clustered low shoddy buildings, the ramshackle bulk of a solar-power trap with auxiliary electricity generator, staff living-quarters, piles of old crates, a small sewage plant, old cars and old bicycles, a goat, an Indian charpoy with a man lying on it, rubbish in black containers, builders' materials, litter.

"You want to get a Crosswell's Tape, honey. That's my secret. Keeps me in trim all the time."

"What's a Crosswell's Tape, for god's sake?"

He winced. Although Zadar Smith World had handled Crosswell's promotion for six-seven years now, this fluff had never heard of their Tape. *And* she worked in Promotion.

"Crosswell's Tape is a worm. A laboratory-mutated version of a beef tapeworm. Thoroughly safe, totally symbiotic, a great little feeder. Only needs replacing once every decade. Lodges in the small intestine, causes no discomfort. Enables you to eat up to fifty percent more *and* keep your figure. Greatest social invention of the century."

"Oh, what they call the slimmer. I never tried one."

Saul's teeth had picked the drumstick clean. He flung it towards the ocean. It fell short and hit the sand.

Behind the hotel was the twenty-foot-high wire barrier cutting the sanctuary off from the rest of India. It ran parallel to the ocean as far as the eye could be bothered to see, in one direction; in the other, it angled off behind the hotel and ran down into the waves. Behind the wire barrier stood or sat solitary figures; sometimes there was a little family group. They all waited patiently in the hot sun, looking at the spot where Saul's bone had fallen. Although there were possibly several hundreds of figures behind the wire, they were motionless and well-spaced, except round the gate, so that the effect was one of solitude, rather than over-crowding.

"Do you think one of those tapes would help my thighs, Sauly?"

She got her camera ready to photograph the Indians behind the barrier. There was a cute little girl just standing there, not a stitch on, about four years old—you couldn't tell her age really—with a cute little fat pot on her. Make a nice picture to take home to the States. They didn't *look* starving, despite all the propaganda.

Their taxi slid up with a Sikh driver at the wheel, luxuriant in beard and green turban. Paidie took a photograph of him instead. The Sikh smiled and opened the car door for her. He was hairy, wow! Saul didn't have any hair at all, not anywhere on his body.

He caught and diagnosed her glance at the driver. "These guys have lousy org-ratings, honey, you know that? This chauffeur guy has probably never rated better than seven in his life. Six, more like."

In perfect English, the Sikh said, "Pardon me, sir, but there are famine riots in the bazaar every day this week. It may be dangerous to go there. All of Kerala is in ferment."

"The Luxor must protect us. Tourists bring in dollars—we're the Luxor's responsibility, right? Are we supposed to stay behind that lousy chicken wire all week?"

"You are in front of it, sir. It is the native population who is behind it. It is there for your protection."

"Well, you protect us in the bazaar. The famine's nothing to do with us. I take it you have a revolver, man?"

"Yes, sir. I always carry a revolver."

"You shoot well?"

"I am a very good shot, sir, or I do not get this job."

"Let's get doing, then. Bazaar, and step on it!"

As the big black car slid through the gates, Saul, prompted by generosity, threw a stick of Lifesavers out of the window. The ragged crowd dived for it. As they scrabbled in the dust, he was reminded of his dream.

"Wonder whose skulls they were? Every dream has to have a meaning. Guess it must have meant I was exploring the unconscious of mankind. You know, honey, I am a kind of genius. I invented the orgasm-rating system."

Paidie was staring through the window, not attending again.

"What a rotten road they have here! Say, Saul, I'd hate to *live* in India, wouldn't you? They're so dirty and poor."

The poor and dirty were pressing close to the car, shouting or waving hands. The Sikh put his sandalled foot down and they bucked along the road.

"They're under-developed, that's why. You know that. Yeah, the org-rating system was my big big contribution to Advertising. Made my name, sold a thousand products. Then the psycho-analytical guys came along and discovered my concept had real bedrock psychological truth behind it! How you like that?"

"Saul, darling, do you really think it is safe here? Suppose your dream was a warning about venturing among primitive people or something?"

"Who wanted to do this anyway—you or me?"

The car drew up under an avenue of tattered deodar trees, where dogs scuttled and people squatted. There were a few stalls here, and shrill music playing. Saul continued his lecture. To hell with local color.

". . . Since when research has proved that there are different levels of sexual enjoyment, just like different levels of sleep. Fert-Asia estimates that eighty-five percent of the population in this area, male and female, never do any better than a grade six orgasm. How'd you like that? Of course, it all stems from infantile malnutrition. And in India alone . . ."

Boredom drove her out of the car. She stood under the trees, a chubby blonde in high-heeled sandals, wearing almost nothing, fresh from hotels, Concordes, and offices all sanitized for her protection. The scarecrows round about her had eyes of coal. They were thin and beautiful and burnished. They all ran to sell her anything they had, melons, brass statues, photos of little girls embracing goats, jewels, clay figurines, dried fish. Paidie fell into a panic, stamping her pretty foot till her breasts trembled.

"Saul, those dream skulls! Suppose they were ours, yours and mine!"

The crowd pressed closer. She hit out with her handbag. One of the beggars touched her. Then they fell on her. Paidie was screaming.

Saul was shaking the Sikh's shoulders. "Shoot, shoot, you lunatic! Fire into the crowd. Or give me the gun!" He was vividly aware of the noise and the heat and the stink.

The Sikh started up the car, backed it swiftly away, turned, raced back for the hotel. "Better not to shoot, sir, or we all get very much trouble. This is great time of trouble, please take my undoubted word!"

Saul sank back into his seat, chewing his lips. "Maybe you're right. The hotel can send out a rescue party for Paidie. She wasn't in my dream. There was just me, dressed up as Jung . . . what the hell was I doing? I hate dreaming about death or all that."

Inside the hotel, it was wonderfully cool and quiet. Saul ordered a Martini to soothe his nerves.

THE TRUTH ABOUT PYECRAFT

by H. G. Wells

He sits not a dozen yards away. If I glance over my shoulder I can see him. And if I catch his eye—and usually I catch his eye—it meets me with an expression——

It is mainly an imploring look—and yet with suspicion in it.

Confound his suspicion! If I wanted to tell on him I should have told long ago. I don't tell and I don't tell, and he ought to feel at his ease. As if anything so gross and fat as he could feel at ease! Who would believe me if I did tell?

Poor old Pyecraft! Great, uneasy jelly of substance! The fattest clubman in London.

He sits at one of the little club tables in the huge bay by the fire, stuffing. What is he stuffing? I glance judiciously and catch him biting at the round of hot buttered teacake, with his eyes on me. Confound him!—with his eyes on me!

That settles it, Pyecraft! Since you *will* be abject, since you *will* behave as though I was not a man of honour, here, right under your embedded eyes, I write the thing down—the plain truth about Pyecraft. The man I helped, the man I shielded, and who has requited me by making my club unendurable, absolutely unendurable, with his liquid appeal, with the perpetual "don't tell" of his looks.

And, besides, why does he keep on eternally eating?

Well, here goes for the truth, the whole truth, and nothing but the truth!

Pyecraft——I made the acquaintance of Pyecraft in this very smoking-room. I was a young, nervous new member, and he saw it. I was sitting all alone, wishing I knew more of the members, and suddenly he came, a great rolling front of chins and abdomina, towards me, and grunted and sat down in a chair close by me and wheezed for a space, and scraped for a space with a match and lit a cigar, and then addressed me. I forget what he said—something about the matches not lighting properly, and afterwards as he talked he kept stopping the waiters one by one as they went by, and telling them about the matches in that thin, fluty voice he has. But, anyhow, it was in some such way we began our talking.

He talked about various things and came round to games. And thence to my figure and complexion. "You ought to be a good cricketer," he said. I suppose I am slender, slender to what some people would call lean, and I suppose I am rather dark, still—— I am not ashamed of having a Hindu great-grandmother, but, for all that, I don't want casual strangers to see through me at a glance to *her*. So that I was set against Pyecraft from the beginning.

But he only talked about me in order to get to himself.

"I expect," he said, "you take no more exercise than I do, and probably you eat no less." (Like all excessively obese people he fancied he ate nothing.) "Yet"—and he smiled an oblique smile—"we differ."

And then he began to talk about his fatness and his fatness; all he did for his fatness and all he was going to do for his fatness; what people had advised him to do for his fatness and what he had heard of people doing for fatness similar to his. "*A priori,*" he said, "one would think a question of nutrition could be answered by dietary and a question of assimilation by drugs." It was stifling. It was dumpling talk. It made me feel swelled to hear him.

One stands that sort of thing once in a way at a club, but a time came when I fancied I was standing too much. He took to me altogether too conspicuously. I could never go into the smoking-room but he would come wallowing towards me, and sometimes he came and gormandised round and about me while I had my lunch. He seemed at times almost to be clinging to me. He was a bore, but not so fearful a bore as to be limited to me; and from the first, there was something in his manner—almost as though he knew, almost as though he penetrated to the fact that I *might*—that there was a remote, exceptional chance in me that no one else presented.

"I'd give anything to get it down," he would say— "anything," and peer at me over his vast cheeks and pant.

Poor old Pyecraft! He has just gonged, no doubt to order another buttered teacake!

He came to the actual thing one day. "Our Pharmacopoeia," he said, "our Western Pharmacopoeia, is anything but the last word of medical science. In the East, I've been told——"

He stopped and stared at me. It was like being at an aquarium.

I was suddenly angry with him. "Look here," I said, "who told you about my great-grandmother's recipes?"

"Well," he fenced.

"Every time we've met for a week," I said—"and we've met pretty often—you've given me a broad hint or so about that little secret of mine."

"Well," he said, "now the cat's out of the bag, I'll admit, yes, it is so. I had it——"

"From Pattison?"

"Indirectly," he said, which I believe was lying, "yes."

"Pattison," I said, "took that stuff at his own risk."

He pursed his mouth and bowed.

"My great-grandmother's recipes," I said, "are queer things to handle. My father was near making me promise——"

"He didn't?"

"No. But he warned me. He himself used one—once."

"Ah! . . . But do you think——? Suppose—suppose there did happen to be one——"

"The things are curious documents," I said. "Even the smell of 'em. . . . No!"

But after going so far Pyecraft was resolved I should go farther. I was always a little afraid if I tried his patience too much he would fall on me suddenly and smother me. I own I was weak. But I was also annoyed with Pyecraft. I had got to that state of feeling for him that disposed me to say, "Well, *take* the risk!" The little affair of Pattison to which I have alluded was a different matter altogether. What it was doesn't concern us now, but I knew, anyhow, that the particular recipe I used then was safe. The rest I didn't know so much about, and, on the whole, I was inclined to doubt their safety pretty completely.

Yet even if Pyecraft got poisoned——

I must confess the poisoning of Pyecraft struck me as an immense undertaking.

That evening I took that queer, odd-scented sandal-wood box out of my safe and turned the rustling skins over. The gentleman who wrote the recipes for my great-grandmother evidently had a weakness for skins of a miscellaneous origin, and his handwriting was cramped to the last degree. Some of the things are quire unreadable to me—though my family, with its Indian Civil Service associations, has kept up a knowledge of Hindustani from generation to generation—and none are absolutely plain sailing. But I found the one that I knew was there soon enough, and sat on the floor by my safe for some time looking at it.

"Look here," said I to Pyecraft next day, and snatched the slip away from his eager grasp.

"So far as I can make it out, this is a recipe for Loss of Weight. ("Ah!" said Pyecraft.) I'm not absolutely sure, but I think it's that. And if you take my advice you'll leave it alone. Because, you know—I blacken my blood in your interest, Pyecraft—my ancestors on that side were, so far as I can gather, a jolly queer lot. See?"

"Let me try it," said Pyecraft.

I leant back in my chair. My imagination made one mighty effort and fell flat within me. "What in Heaven's name, Pyecraft," I asked, "do you think you'll look like when you get thin?"

He was impervious to reason. I made him promise never to say a word to me about his disgusting fatness again whatever happened—never, and then I handed him that little piece of skin.

"It's nasty stuff," I said.

"No matter," he said, and took it.

He goggled at it. "But—but——" he said.

He had just discovered that it wasn't English.

"To the best of my ability," I said, "I will do you a translation."

I did my best. After that we didn't speak for a fortnight. Whenever he approached me I frowned and motioned him away, and he respected our compact, but at the end of the fortnight he was as fat as ever. And then he got a word in.

"I must speak," he said. "It isn't fair. There's something wrong. It's done me no good. You're not doing your great-grandmother justice."

"Where's the recipe?"

He produced it gingerly from his pocket-book.

I ran my eye over the items. "Was the egg addled?" I asked.

"No. Ought it to have been?"

"That," I said, "goes without saying in all my poor dear great-grandmother's recipes. When condition or quality is not specified you must get the worst. She was drastic or nothing. . . . And there's one or two possible alternatives to some of these other things. You got *fresh* rattlesnake venom?"

"I got rattlesnake from Jamrach's. It cost—it cost——"

"That's your affair, anyhow. This last item——"

"I know a man who——"

"Yes. H'm. Well, I'll write the alternatives down. So far as I know the language, the spelling of this recipe is particu- larly atrocious. By-the-bye, dog here probably means pa- riah dog."

For a month after that I saw Pyecraft constantly at the club and as fat and anxious as ever. He kept our treaty, but at times he broke the spirit of it by shaking his head despondently. Then one day in the cloak-room he said, "Your great-grandmother——"

"Not a word against her," I said: and he held his peace.

I could have fancied he had desisted, and I saw him one day talking to three new members about his fatness as though he was in search of other recipes. And then, quite unexpectedly his telegram came.

"Mr. Formalyn!" bawled a page-boy under my nose and I took the telegram and opened it at once.

"For Heaven's sake come.—Pyecraft."

"H'm," said I, and to tell the truth I was so pleased at the rehabilitation of my great-grandmother's reputation this evidently promised that I made a most excellent lunch.

I got Pyecraft's address from the hall porter. Pyecraft inhabited the upper half of a house in Bloomsbury, and I went there as soon as I had done my coffee and Trappistine. I did not wait to finish my cigar.

"Mr. Pyecraft?" said I, at the front door.

They believed he was ill; he hadn't been out for two days.

"He expects me," said I, and they sent me up.

I rang the bell at the lattice-door upon the landing.

"He shouldn't have tried it, anyhow," I said to myself. "A man who eats like a pig ought to look like a pig."

An obviously worthy woman, with an anxious face and a carelessly placed cap, came and surveyed me through the lattice.

I gave my name and she opened his door for me in a dubious fashion.

"Well?" said I, as we stood together inside Pyecraft's piece of the landing.

" 'E said you was to come in if you came," she said, and regarded me, making no motion to show me anywhere. And then, confidentially, " 'e's locked in, sir."

"Locked in?"

"Locked himself in yesterday morning and 'asn't let anyone in since, sir. And ever and again *swearing.* Oh, my!"

I stared at the door she indicated by her glances. "In there?" I said.

"Yes, sir."

"What's up?"

She shook her head sadly. " 'E keeps on calling for vittles, sir. *'Eavy* vittles 'e wants. I get 'im what I can. Pork 'e's 'ad, sooit puddin', sossiges, noo bread. Everythink like that. Left outside, if you please, and me go away. 'E's eatin' sir, somethink *awful*."

There came a piping bawl from inside the door: "That Formalyn?"

"That you, Pyecraft?" I shouted, and went and banged the door.

"Tell her to go away."

I did.

Then I could hear a curious pattering upon the door, almost like someone feeling for the handle in the dark, and Pyecraft's familiar grunts.

"It's all right," I said, "she's gone."

But for a long time the door didn't open.

I heard the key turn. Then Pyecraft's voice said, "Come in."

I turned the handle and opened the door. Naturally I expected to see Pyecraft.

Well, you know, he wasn't there!

I never had such a shock in my life. There was his sitting-room in a state of untidy disorder, plates and dishes among the books and writing things, and several chairs overturned, but Pyecraft——

"It's all right, o' man; shut the door," he said, and then I discovered him.

There he was right up close to the cornice in the corner by the door, as though someone had glued him to the ceiling. His face was anxious and angry. He panted and gesticulated. "Shut the door," he said. "If that woman gets hold of it——"

I shut the door, and went and stood away from him and stared.

"If anything gives way and you tumble down," I said, "you'll break your neck, Pyecraft."

"I wish I could," he wheezed.

"A man of your age and weight getting up to kiddish gymnastics——"

"Don't," he said and looked agonized. "Your damned great-grandmother——"

"Be careful," I warned him.

"I'll tell you," he said, and gesticulated.

"How the deuce," said I, "are you holding on up there?"

And then abruptly I realized that he was not holding on at all, that he was floating up there—just as a gas-filled bladder might have floated in the same position. He began a struggle to thrust himself away from the ceiling and to clamber down the wall to me. "It's that prescription," he panted, as he did so. "Your great-gran——"

"*No!*" I cried.

He took hold of a framed engraving rather carelessly as he spoke and it gave way, and he flew back to the ceiling again, while the picture smashed on to the sofa. Bump he went against the ceiling, and I knew then why he was all over white on the more salient curves and angles of his person. He tried again more carefully, coming down by way of the mantel.

It was really a most extraordinary spectacle, that great, fat, apoplectic-looking man upside down and trying to get from the ceiling to the floor. "That prescription," he said. "Too successful."

"How?"

"Loss of weight—almost complete."

And then, of course, I understood.

"By Jove, Pyecraft," said I, "what you wanted was a cure for fatness! But you always called it weight. You would call it weight."

Somehow I was extremely delighted. I quite liked Pyecraft for the time. "Let me help you!" I said, and took his hand and pulled him down. He kicked about, trying to get foothold somewhere. It was very like holding a flag on a windy day.

"That table," he said, pointing, "is solid mahogany and very heavy. If you can put me under that——"

I did, and there he wallowed about like a captive balloon, while I stood on his hearthrug and talked to him.

I lit a cigar. "Tell me," I said, "what happened?"

"I took it," he said.

"How did it taste?"

"Oh, *beastly!*"

I should fancy they all did. Whether one regards the ingredients or the probable compound or the possible results, almost all my great-grandmother's remedies appear to me at least to be extraordinarily uninviting. For my own part——

"I took a little sip first."

"Yes?"

"And as I felt light and better after an hour, I decided to take the draught."

"My dear Pyecraft!"

"I held my nose," he explained. "And then I kept on getting lighter and lighter—and helpless, you know."

He gave way suddenly to a burst of passion. "What the goodness am I to *do?*" he said.

"There's one thing pretty evident," I said, "that you mustn't do. If you go out of doors you'll go up and up." I waved an arm upward. "They'd have to send Santos-Dumont after you to bring you down again."

"I suppose it will wear off?"

I shook my head. "I don't think you can count on that," I said.

And then there was another burst of passion, and he kicked out at adjacent chairs and banged the floor. He behaved just as I should have expected a great, fat, self-indulgent man to behave under trying circumstances—that is to say, very badly. He spoke of me and of my great-grandmother with an utter want of discretion.

"I never asked you to take the stuff," I said.

And generously disregarding the insults he was putting upon me, I sat down in his armchair and began to talk to him in a sober, friendly fashion.

I pointed out to him that this was a trouble he had brought upon himself, and that it had almost an air of poetical justice. He had eaten too much. This he disputed, and for a time we argued the point.

He became noisy and violent, so I desisted from this aspect of his lesson. "And then," said I, "you committed the sin of euphuism. You called it, not Fat, which is just and inglorious, but Weight. You——"

He interrupted to say that he recognised all that. What was he to *do?*

I suggested he should adapt himself to his new conditions. So we came to the really sensible part of the business. I suggested that it would not be difficult for him to learn to walk about on the ceiling with his hands——

"I can't sleep," he said.

But that was no great difficulty. It was quite possible, I pointed out, to make a shake-up under a wire mattress, fasten the under things on with wire tapes, and have a blanket, sheet, and coverlid to button at the side. He would have to confide in his housekeeper, I said; and after some squabbling he agreed to that. (Afterwards it was quite delightful to see the beautifully matter-of-fact way with which the good lady took all these amazing inversions.) He could have a library ladder in his room, and all his meals could be laid on the top of his bookcase. We also hit on an ingenious device by which he could get to the floor whenever he wanted, which was simply to put the *British Encyclopaedia* (tenth edition) on top of his open shelves. He just pulled out a couple of volumes and held on, and down he came. And we agreed there must be iron staples along the skirting, so that he could cling to those whenever he wanted to get about the room on the lower level.

As we got on with the thing I found myself almost keenly interested. It was I who called in the housekeeper and broke matters to her, and it was I chiefly who fixed up the inverted bed. In fact, I spent two whole days at his flat. I am a handy, interfering sort of man with a screwdriver, and I made all sorts of ingenious adaptations for him—ran a wire to bring his bells within reach, turned all his electric lights up instead of down, and so on. The whole affair was extremely curious and interesting to me, and it was delightful to think of Pyecraft like some great, fat blow-fly, crawling about on his ceiling and clambering round the lintel of his doors from one room to another, and never, never, never coming to the club any more. . . .

Then, you know, my fatal ingenuity got the better of me. I was sitting by his fire drinking his whisky, and he was up in his favourite corner by the cornice, tacking a Turkey carpet to the ceiling, when the idea struck me. "By Jove, Pyecraft!" I said, "all this is totally unnecessary."

And before I could calculate the complete consequences of my notion I blurted it out. "Lead underclothing," said I, and the mischief was one.

Pyecraft received the thing almost in tears. "To be right ways up again—" he said.

I gave him the whole secret before I saw where it would take me. "Buy sheet lead," I said, "stamp it into discs. Sew 'em all over your underclothes until you have enough. Have lead-soled boots, carry a bag of solid lead, and the thing is done! Instead of being a prisoner here you may go abroad again, Pyecraft! you may travel——"

A still happier idea came to me. "You need never fear a shipwreck. All you need do is just slip off some or all of your clothes, take the necessary amount of luggage in your hand, and float up in the air——"

In his emotion he dropped the tack-hammer within an ace of my head. "By Jove!" he said, "I shall be able to come back to the club again."

The thing pulled me up short. "By Jove!" I said, faintly. "Yes. Of course—you will."

He did. He does. There he sits behind me now stuffing—as I live!—a third go of buttered teacake. And no one in the whole world knows—except his housekeeper and

In his emotion he dropped the tack-hammer within an ace of my head. "By Jove!" he said, "I shall be able to come back to the club again."

The thing pulled me up short. "By Jove!" I said, faintly. "Yes. Of course—you will."

He did. He does. There he sits behind me now stuffing—as I live!—a third go of buttered teacake. And no one in the whole world knows—except his housekeeper and me—that he weighs practically nothing; that he is a mere boring mass of assimilatory matters, mere clouds in clothing, *niente, nefas,* and most inconsiderable of men. There he sits watching until I have done this writing. Then, if he can, he will waylay me. He will come billowing up to me...

He will tell me over again all about it, how it feels, how it doesn't feel, how he sometimes hopes it is passing off a little. And always somewhere in that fat, abundant discourse he will say, "The secret's keeping, eh? If anyone knew of it—I should be so ashamed. . . . Makes a fellow look such a fool, you know. Crawling about a ceiling and all that. . . ."

And now to elude Pyecraft, occupying, as he does, an admirable strategic position between me and the door.